YIN Ain't YANG

The Ancient Way to Better Health

Lester Sawicki DDS

www.Tooth-Fight.com
www.Teethsense.com
www.Revolutiontooth.com
info@revolutiontooth.com

Library of Congress Control Number: 2012900560
ISBN: 9780984370658

Interior Design by William Groetzinger

Also by Lester Sawicki, DDS

Reflections On A Smile
The Teeth Whitening Cure
Teeth In Mortal Combat
The Tao of Tooth

YIN Ain't YANG

The Ancient Way to Better Health

BONUS BOOK
Teeth In Mortal Combat
How to Unleash Your Basic Instinct For Survival

BONUS CHAPTERS: PART 1
Teeth In Mortal Combat

BONUS CHAPTERS: PART 2
The Teeth Whitening Cure

Yoga unites the 3 treasures of tai chi

beauty, love, spirit,

*however, joining the upper and lower teeth
is the simplest path to understanding.*

—*from the TAO TE TOOTH*

YIN Ain't YANG

The Ancient Way
to Better Health

Lester Sawicki DDS

CHAPTER 1
BOOST YOUR CHAKRAS
WITH TEETH CHI ENERGY

Teeth Chi Energy To Vitalize The Body's Chakras

Through my practices of dentistry and martial arts I discovered compelling evidence regarding the vital importance of teeth to human survival, and learned that by strengthening the Qi (vital life force) of the oral cavity one can significantly boost jawbone mineral density, protect teeth from occlusal stress fractures, restore and enhance periodontal health, alleviate TMJ dysfunction, increase blood flow to the brain, improve overall body balance and muscular strength, and accelerate thought processes. Training the teeth, tongue and jaw increases salivary flow, which releases a surge of insulin thereby increasing heart rate and sending glucose and oxygen to the brain to help us learn faster and retain information longer. Cerebrospinal fluid flow to the prefrontal cortex is facilitated, thereby strengthening the body's natural protection against addictions.

The mouth remains a potent, albeit unused, weapon of self-defense today. It is a reservoir of powerful Qi that can be used to access and strengthen the body's chakras (vital energy centers) to ensure a long, healthy and prosperous life. The book *Teeth in Mortal Combat: How to Unleash your Basic Instinct for Survival* illuminates the importance of teeth not only as a weapon, but as a key to boosting one's overall health and fitness as well as understanding our place in the cosmos.

I believe this information is invaluable to dentists. As the future "Masters of Holistic Health," we can use our levelheaded common sense and influence to instruct our patients—both young and old—on the value of maintaining and enhancing tooth function beyond ordinary use into the realm of the extraordinary: 32 precious pearls of life that immeasurably affect one's happiness and enable the fulfillment of one's destiny.

An ever-increasing number of dentists are becoming concerned that current dental marketing oversells the simplistic and often unrealistic nature of cosmetic dentistry: artificially whitened teeth are essential to creating the sexually attractive smile that makes all dreams come true. This marketing conceit completely overshadows the notion of any real connection between strong, functional teeth and one's overall health and longevity.

Modern science is just now catching up to the ancient understanding of this link between a healthy oral cavity and general health and longevity. The knowledge that the teeth are joined to vital organs by way of the energy channels (internal pathways of Qi) has been known for thousands of years. Likewise, the self-healing properties of the teeth were known to the ancients. And the awareness that it is possible to energetically strengthen the teeth, tongue and jaw beyond what is considered normal is thousands of years old.

The energy exercises revealed in the book are most appropriately taught and experienced outside of the traditional model of dental care in a peaceful, meditative environment away from stress-inducing dental offices. Of course the most effective way for dentists to enrich the lives of their patients is to focus on our specialty—restoration of the oral cavity—and also to be a living testament to the value of maintaining and strengthening the teeth, tongue and jaw.

Patients need to be willing to commit a small amount of personal time each day to these exercises. Five or 10 additional minutes tacked on to one's daily exercise regimen is not too much for most people. A few of the exercises are simple enough for people to learn from the book, but there are, of course, advantages to personal instruction.

I had an interesting experience a short time after I began this training. By merely visualizing the act of chewing gum, I was able to 'feel' the chewy resistance of the gum and the accompanying salivary secretions. My focus improved, breathing became fuller and deeper, and I felt simultaneously relaxed and revitalized.

This through-the-looking-glass awareness and tactile familiarity with the structures within the oral cavity led me to a humbling respect for the teeth, tongue and jaw and their relation to me in my roles as human, martial artist and dentist.

A dental school classmate invited me to join his evening kung fu exercise program. Later he suggested I come to his Tai Chi Master's introductory seminar where I witnessed physical and energetic feats way beyond my normal awareness and experience. That was more than 30 years ago and I'm still enthusiastically searching for and studying new theories of personal development.

One of the best places to begin personal instruction in teeth training is with the "Fit 150—Intended Evolution" organization.

CHAPTER 2
FITNESS FOR YOUR TEETH —WHO'D A THOUGHT!
By Teresa Mullan Frease, M-Phil

Fitness training for your teeth!?!? This, coupled with intention, is incorporated into a brand new approach to fitness and health. Intended Evolution Fitness, or Fit-150, is a new scientifically-based, revolutionary approach to health and fitness. It combines exercises from the Eastern traditional health arts with the power of "Intention" and the mind. Dr. Dongxun Zhang, founder of FIT-150, is a doctor of Oriental medicine and Acupuncture, as well as a renowned Qigong and Tai Chi Master. His theory of Intended Evolution contends that conscious intention actively shapes your health. He believes the mind is very powerful and if used along with physical exercise, this power can generate great benefits for your health and longevity. Many people have limiting beliefs about aging. However, Fit-150 believes the mind has the power to actually realign cellular memory so that we can no longer be negatively impacted by these limiting beliefs about aging. FIT-150 teaches us to break out of these beliefs and to create the life and health that is our birthright! For multiple generations our teeth and jaws have been degenerating. This is largely due to the quality and types of food the mass population consumes. Teeth are no longer challenged and used in as many different ways as in the past. Dr Zhang believes food today is largely processed and hence does not provide the necessary challenge to the teeth and jaws to keep them strong and healthy. He believes this degeneration of the jaw and related muscles may also affect other areas close by such as the nose and eyes. Dental health is also very important for digestion and related functions. It is a very important part of the health of the whole body. FIT-150 recommends that to maintain optimal dental health, some challenge is necessary to the teeth and jaws to function more in line with their original purpose. This is the "Use it or lose it theory". FIT-150 teaches exercises for the teeth and jaws and how to create a "blueprint" to keep them healthy and strong. This is designed to keep them strong all the way to the grand age of 150 years old!!…If you plan to live that long. Positively planning to "live that long" is exactly what Fit-150 recommends you do! Learning how to establish a blueprint for the health of your teeth is similar to building a foundation to support a 10-story building. Even if the actual building ends up being only 4-stories, we know the foundation built for 10-stories will easily support this. Regardless if you live to 80, 100 or 150, FIT-150 creates a blueprint for your teeth to be healthy throughout your entire life. FIT-150 not only addresses dental health but goes beyond this to provide cardiovascular and flexibility training. It integrates specific exercises, techniques and intentions for increased bone density, hormonal balance, lymph circulation, organ detoxification, brain function, sexual health and overall happiness of the mind, body and spirit. Exercise your mind and teeth and live happily all the way to 150 as you enjoy the health and vitality of all aspects of your body's functioning!

CHAPTER 3

NOW THERE'S A NEW MARTIAL ARTS BOOK THAT REVEALS TOOTH AND JAW STRENGTHENING EXERCISES FOR HEALTH, LONGEVITY AND BASIC SURVIVAL INSTINCTS.

Teeth in Mortal Combat: How to Unleash Your Basic Instinct for Survival examines the role teeth play in activating primitive instincts for martial arts, health and longevity. It seeks to reveal how the teeth and jaw are powerful tools that not only can serve as survival weapons but can also unlock vital life energy that may improve overall health. The origins of self-defense relied on basic weapons—sharp teeth and strong jaws. In my decades of experience as practicing dentist and martial artist, I believe that focus on the strength and purpose of the mouth in relation to the rest of the body's survival has been neglected. In *Teeth in Mortal Combat,* the idea is presented that enhancing the chi, or life energy, of the mouth may significantly boost jawbone mineral density, increase blood flow to the brain, and improve overall balance and muscular strength. *Teeth in Mortal Combat* is intended for martial artists, yoga practitioners, meditation students, dental professionals, as well as the general public. The book offers a series of energy-building exercises aimed at strengthening and aligning the chi center of the oral cavity with the power centers of the body. Practicing these exercises can lead to a deeper understanding of man's place in the cosmos and boost one's overall health and fitness. *Teeth in Mortal Combat* is available online at *Amazon.com* and other channels.

CHAPTER 4
WHAT IS TOOTH MEDITATION?

If you are looking to feel healthy and fit, while extending your lifespan, then Tooth Meditation might be for you. Quiet meditation alone can help for a while, but that could take your energy away from the path of longevity. Tooth Meditation helps build your energy and move it in your body because longevity is all about movement, everything flowing and moving in a circle. The easiest way to get your energy flowing is to involve the physical body.

Tooth Meditation is more than physical fitness for your teeth and jaws. It's actually mental and physical. It builds inner strength by boosting your brain power and it builds your outer physical body. It strengthens your teeth, jaws, joints, muscles, and tendons, particularly in your jaw and neck area, your shoulders, your spine, your inner organs, your breathing, and your focus. It's the physical movement and mental drive which enhances your health by releasing stuck and stagnant energy that leads to disease.

Tooth Meditation might be the single most profound, life changing experience you'll ever come across.

CHAPTER 5
MEDITATION CAN BE COMPLICATED BUT NOT WITH THIS CALMING DENTAL MAGIC

Basic Tooth Wiggle Meditation

Tooth exercise combined with meditation is important if you're serious about increasing your fitness, health and vitality. All the meridians of the body eventually flow through the teeth. And when it comes to preventing oral health problems…3 IS THE MAGIC NUMBER!… Teeth, Gums, Bone. In addition to a toothbrush and floss, tooth meditation can be your best friend. Any weakness in the teeth, gums, and jawbone can lead to a disruption of the flow of your chi (energy) to practically every organ in your body. Any kink in your oral streams of chi may develop into physical weakness, mental impairment, and shortened life span. Maintaining strong, healthy and functional teeth and gums is vital to overall fitness and health. You can learn more on the subject by visiting *www.Tooth-Fight.com* and *www.Revolutiontooth. com*. Here's a simple tooth meditation to get you started in the right direction:

Sit upright in a chair. Imagine yourself a magnificent tall green pine tree, flexible but rooted firm and steady against the forces of nature. You can start with any molar—top/bottom and right or left. Take your index finger and press on the outside of the very last molar in your mouth. Then slightly release the pressure as the tip of your tongue presses firmly on the inside of the tooth. Wiggle the tooth between your finger and tongue. If the tip of your tongue cannot reach the last molar then you may have a condition called "tongue tie" and it would be wise to consult with your dentist to see if it can be surgically corrected.

The tongue is a powerful conduit of energy. Chinese medical theory believes it is an extension of the heart and you can imagine all the varied ways your tongue's power points outward to the world around you. Since the average person pays little attention to his teeth your finger is used to locate the tooth and to help focus your attention on it while your mind activates the tongue to fill your tooth and surrounding bone with light energy.

Slowly and alternately press with finger and tip of tongue to wiggle the tooth. Inhale when you press with your finger. Slowly exhale the grounded energy out of the tip of your tongue into the tooth as your tongue presses the tooth firmly. Relax the tongue and press the finger as you inhale, then relax the finger and push the tooth with the tip of the tongue as you slowly exhale through the tongue into the tooth.

This is a slow, relaxed, meditative exercise to fill your tooth and surrounding bone with light energy. On the exhale imagine and feel the tooth expanding as a balloon and see the light coming through your tongue into the tooth filling the balloon with a high intensity glow. Gradually the glow extends down the root of the tooth and finally infiltrates outward into the surrounding jawbone.

After a couple of breaths move to the adjacent tooth and repeat the steps. This meditative exercise can be mentally tiring for beginners so stop after you reach your front tooth, usually no more than 8 teeth during a session. It is recommended you concentrate on only one quadrant or quarter of your mouth at each session. You need practice this only once or twice a week to reap invaluable benefits.

CHAPTER 6
PULL A TOOTH, LOSE A BRAIN CELL?

Japanese and Swedish researchers observed that elderly mice, monkeys and people have difficulty with short term memory after all the teeth are pulled. The link between teeth and memory loss was noted only in the old aged and no conclusion has been reached as to the reason.

Some believe that chewing with teeth increases blood circulation in the head and neck bringing oxygen-rich blood to the brain. The more teeth one has the more likely one is to chew with a greater number of chomps per mouthful resulting in greater oxygenation and less risk of dementia. Chewing gum is now recommended for German school children to help improve learning. The military has long ago given out free gum to keep the ranks more alert.

Another possibility is that gum disease infection is the most common cause of tooth loss in the elderly and the release of inflammatory substances into the brain may cause brain neuron death in an old body that is already compromised with age related dysfunctions.

And some think that chewing sends signals to certain brain regions which in turn reduces stress hormone levels in the blood. If older people can't chew their stress levels might rise enough to cause brain impairment for short term memory. Luckily this problem is not usually seen in young or middle age people and mice.

Chinese traditional medicine has a theory which connects the teeth with the brain. You can learn more at Jade Spirit Community Acupuncture in Phoenix, Arizona.

You should be warned that what we have so far are theories and there is no proven link between chewing, tooth loss and dementia. Your teeth are, however, critical to complete mastication and efficient digestion of food to help the body fully utilize their nutrients. It would be prudent to preserve and maintain healthy teeth if only to enjoy your favorite treats and prevent aromatic wind from poorly digested food. Remember, there might be a good reason why the third molars have been traditionally called "wisdom teeth!"

Chapter 7

YOU CAN SLAM THE BRAKES ON HARMFUL UNCONSCIOUS TOOTH GRINDING WITH THESE FREE, EASY TO DO EXERCISES.

A common question is whether there is a meditation to help with harmful habitual unconscious teeth grinding. My puppy dog, Scary Plodder, helped me answer this. Scary has chattering teeth. :(So I decided to explore chattering in animals before revealing answers for the human condition.

Google "teeth chattering" and you'll find that it is a kind of tremor or involuntary rhythmic muscle contraction and relaxation. in rats it's a sign of pleasure but they also chatter when scared. Maybe you can find glimpses of that rat trait portrayed somewhere between *Willard* (2003) and *Ratatouille* (2007) but it was my own chattering teeth I heard during scenes of terror and amusement.

Considering the wide range of scientific experimentation done with rats you might expect the poor lab rodent to develop paranoid schizophrenic disorders such as teeth grinding or bruxism from the fear or pleasure it vicariously experiences as it observes drug testing and surgical/chemical mutilation on its rat partners in the cage. But no, teeth chattering is considered a normal genetic feature of rats that probably evolved over millions of years to help control the length of their open-rooted incisor teeth which means they grow throughout life.

Chattering teeth has a long list of causes most notably thermogenic shivering or cold temperature related conditions. Note that a medical fever without any significant cold exposure can also cause shivering. Chattering can be related with anxiety, extreme fear, seizures, neurologic symptoms of chemical overdose or sensitivity and neurogenic tremors.

If you live with a cat you might notice that its jaws sound a rapid judder or quiver when if stares at a bird through the window. This is more an exaggerated frustrated and uncontrolled shaking of its jaws knowing the glass is a barrier to pouncing on a tasty bird with its vicious killing bite.

Scary Plodder, my cute thin-skinned pup, is a perfect example of canine teeth chattering when very nervous or excited and sometimes with fear. I'm constantly checking her teeth for breaks and cracks. If she doesn't outgrow the condition I'm concerned that with time her chattering will result in excessive wear and tear with permanent damage to her teeth. I rely on my veterinarian to give me advice on how to deal with Scary's chatter.

Human teeth clenching, grinding also known as bruxism is my field of study. Bite protector splints or night guards are the conventional treatment of choice by many dentists but I prefer to try a more holistic approach first. Sleeping with and/or daytime use of a plastic horseshoe like device that snaps over your teeth isn't well accepted by most of my patients. Believe me. From my personal experience wearing a night guard splint is more than a clumsy mouthful.

If you've been advised to wear a night guard for excessive bruxism then you might want to try the following meditative exercise first to help alleviate the condition. You should know there is a nutritional factor which won't be talked about here. In most cases I find it too difficult to isolate a vitamin deficiency and people end up spending hard earned money on supplements that won't work. Since the facial and chewing muscles are mostly fast twitch type this meditation exercise takes fast twitch to another level. Fast twitch muscles are critical to stable physical balance. They keep you from slipping, tripping and falling head over heals. After about age 35 humans steadily lose functional fast twitch muscle reflex response. If nothing is done to reverse this pattern then by age 65 there is a high incidence of debilitating falls resulting in broken hips and wrists.

The biting and chewing mechanism is also perfectly balanced by nature with fast twitch muscle groups and in order to reduce the disharmony of abnormal teeth grinding, for whatever reason, it's necessary to restore fast twitch balance to the face, head, neck and jaw muscle physiology.

Here's a meditative exercise you can try if clenching and grinding is brought to your attention by your dentist:

1) **This exercise may make you drowsy so you should not try it while controlling heavy machinery including cars and motorbikes.** The best place to do this is while riding as a passenger in a car or bus. The next best place would be a vibrating easy chair, sofa or bed paying special attention to not fall asleep. You can also do this at anytime in a non-vibrating environment, however, better results come with sitting comfortably in a chair.

2) **Relax completely head to toe.** The lips lightly touch limiting your breathing to only the nose. The tongue lightly touches the roof of the mouth. The teeth are touching while not touching meaning there is a very slight space between the upper and lower teeth which is difficult to consciously hold.

3) **Begin your breathing inhale through your nose and fill up your lungs from bottom to top.** Start a slow long inhale with your focus on the lower abdomen slightly expanding out and as the lungs fill up you'll feel your shoulders stretch out and back a little. At this point hold your breath a second while you swallow

some saliva. Then exhale slowly out your nose. At this point swallow a little saliva again before you begin your next inhale. In your mind count out the seconds it takes to inhale completely as well as the number of seconds it takes to exhale. After several repetitions you will likely run out of saliva so at that point continue without making an effort to swallow. After you master this style of breathing you can then Imagine breathing in and out through a thin straw held between your closed lips. Repeat with each complete breath.

4) **Pay special attention to relaxing your facial muscles including eyes, nose, cheeks, lips and jaw.** First in the vibrating environment relax your jaws and feel your teeth barely chatter against each other. Then (in all environments) in a relaxed way, work your fast twitch jaw muscles to click your teeth as lightly and quickly as possible. Keep relaxing into deeper states and allow your teeth to tap and chatter as lightly as possible. If the environment isn't vibrating you'll have to play a greater intentional role working your fast twitch muscles. You might notice normal typical meditative feelings such as the lips swelling, tongue tingling or a tiny bit of pressure building up in your chest or head. These are good signs that your energy is flowing freely through various channels of the body.

There is no time limit on how long to practice this exercise but you'll see benefits more quickly if you focus on it several or more times a day. It will help you learn to relax your nervous system plus retrain your muscles to gently touch the teeth rather than continue heavy clenching and grinding. Eventually you should reduce the amount of time spent in pathologic bruxing, the light chattering will stop and you'll understand the great pleasure reward of being in a balanced peaceful drifting state of mind breathing like a sleeping baby in a rocking cradle.

CHAPTER 8
TOOTH MEDITATION AND BASIC TONGUE POSITION

The most common tongue position for Eastern Tooth Meditation is where the tip of the tongue touches and rests against the palate behind the upper front teeth. There are various reasons for doing this the most popular being that this juncture connects the main upward and downward flowing (yin-yang) meridians which supports healthy free circulating energy. Some meditation teachers accept the radical belief that without the connection intact your rising fire builds up in your brain leading to uncontrolled terrifying visions, beast-like lunacy, and a general problem of mental instability making it difficult to lead a normal life in society.

Esoteric teachings also say that when you are in the proper stillness of meditation, with the tongue touching the palate, a pearl of life filled with honey nectar forms in your mouth and you can swallow, store, and accumulate it into your lower tan-tien to achieve immortality. No one has been able to prove immortality, however, all anecdotal evidence points to certain pleasures experienced during meditation one of which is an infantile blissful oral memory and feeling of breast feeding.

"The 'Anatomy' of Infant Sucking", by Michael W. Woolridge (http://www.health-e-learning.com/resources/articles), states that "The erotic feeling of sucking, whether it be a lollipop, water bottle or beer or some aspect of the anatomy like a nipple, thumb or lingam (phallus in Sanskrit), was developed during infancy to not only create a sensory experience while eating but to provide intimacy training for the child and mother (or primary care giver).

Both the mother and the child produce the 'bonding' neurohormone Oxytocin during nursing."

According to Wikipedia: "Oxytocin is best known for its roles in female reproduction. It is released in large amounts 1) after distension of the cervix and uterus during labor, and 2) after stimulation of the nipples, facilitating birth and breastfeeding. Recent studies have begun to investigate oxytocin's role in various behaviors, including orgasm, social recognition, pair bonding, anxiety, and maternal behaviors. For this reason, it is sometimes referred to as the 'love hormone." (http://en.wikipedia.org/wiki/Oxytocin)

Another interesting article discussing the sexual aspects of tongue and upper palate can be accessed at the blog post : "The upper palate area is filled with nerve endings" (http://www.huffingtonpost.com/suzie-heumann/the-curious-association-o_b_274342.html). These scientific discoveries are significant for practitioners of meditation to help them gain a greater understanding of the physical benefits of daily practice not commonly known to the ancient ones.

Basic tooth meditation instruction includes these steps:

The tip of the tongue rests on the palate behind the front teeth.

The teeth and lips lightly touch.

Breathe through your nose.

Imagine your saliva as a bright sun and swallow it down to your lower tan-tien.

As you practice you'll become aware of and try to recreate the following experiences:

The tongue compresses gently against the palate.

Saliva is secreted automatically.

Negative suction pressure is created to close the circuit for oxytocin release.

Tongue elevation brings the liquid toward the soft palate triggering the swallowing reflex.

Further analysis reveals that the tongue compresses against the palate in a childlike way and remembers that the application of positive pressure on mother's nipple by the surface of the tongue was the primary force to expel milk from her breast. Evidence, largely by analogy from comparative animal studies, suggests that spiked release of oxytocin from the posterior pituitary causes its level in the blood to pass a threshold at which it acts upon its trigger organ—the breasts—triggering the myo-epithelial cells to contract. (During meditation one doesn't imagine a nipple.)

The 'sucking reflex' is elicited by stimulation (tactile/chemical) of the palate by the nipple. As an adult, the mere act of touching the tongue to the sensory nerve plexus on the tissue behind the top front teeth invokes automatic reflexes that secrete saliva. It's a resourceful mechanism that mimics the anatomy and physiology of infant sucking to induce the flow of breast milk into the mouth. It also feels good and helps one to self-induce a state of relaxation.

The question still remains: beyond self-pleasure, what is the value of tongue position during meditation?

Let's first try to develop a theory from a mechanical point of view and then see how this relates with less visible energetic possibilities. This a reverse investigation as the ancient texts read, matter and energy are one but first you have thought energy followed by its physical manifestation.

The standard medical model, imbibed by clinicians and public alike, is the human body as machine. The truth is very different—we're organisms who internally replace ourselves extraordinarily rapidly—with most of us gone within four weeks. Yes, your teeth and bones last a long time, but internally life is light-speed fast—much of the business life of cells resides in proteins and they're gone in hours to days.

The human body regenerates—remakes itself—very quickly, and differently with each change. Nutrients in food, air, and water are needed to feed the cellular engines that make growth and regeneration possible. After birth, the infant's placental connection to it's nutrient food source is cut and the mother's breast nipple becomes the stage where energy intake for rapid growth occurs.

What you have read so far is a simple account of the mechanisms by which a baby removes milk from the breast for sustenance and where, as an adult, your saliva is secreted with oral stimulation and early breastfeeding memory. Like breast milk, saliva has biochemical components and properties important to health:

Anti-Bacterial

Anti-Viral

Anti-Fungal

Buffering

Digestion

Mineralization

Lubrication & viscol-elasticity

Tissue Coating

In summary, resting the tip of your tongue on the palate stimulates salivary secretions and swallowing your saliva during meditation is a natural way to recycle its physical life supporting properties. Stretch your mind another inch and consider your oral sucking anatomy as an esoteric way to enhance and purify your physical/energetic life force body through cultivation of the mystical pearl of immortality.

CHAPTER 9
TOOTH MEDITATION AT YOUR COMPUTER

If you are new to Tooth Meditation then I would like to touch upon some easy-to-do basic elements which can be practiced right in front of your computer.

Part One
A. HYDRATE

Water comprises more of the brain (with estimates of 90%) than of any other organ of the body. Drink some warm water or herbal tea before, during and after meditation to help "keep the wheel greased." Drinking water is very important before any meditation!—as we tend to perspire under stress and trying to relax during meditation can be a challenge for most of us, plus dehydration can effect our concentration negatively

B. POSITION

This is perfect for taking a stress break from your computer.

Sit at the edge of a chair with your spine erect, upper chest slightly puffed out, and chin gently tucked in. Keep your neck and shoulders relatively relaxed. The lips are lightly touching-closed and breathe in and out through you nose. Touch the tip of the tongue to the roof of the mouth. Keep your top and bottom teeth very lightly touching. Relax the face, lips, eye lids, arms legs.

Cross the right leg ankle over the left knee and let it rest there.

Take your right wrist and cross it over the left wrist and link up the fingers so that the right wrist is on top.

Bend the elbows out and gently turn the fingers in towards the body until they rest on the sternum (breast bone) in the center of the chest. Stay in this position.

Keep the ankles crossed and the wrists crossed and then breathe relaxed and evenly in this position for a few minutes. Try to keep your body from swaying as if you are a bamboo tree holding it's roots against the wind. You will be noticeably calmer after that time.

Focus your attention on your teeth and relax the gum tissues around them and the pulp nerve/blood vessels within. You can pay attention to only one tooth or choose several or all of them. Don't forget your wisdom teeth, especially if they have been pulled. The memory of your lost wisdom teeth remains in your jawbone and you should pay them respect.

When you feel yourself begin to tire in the sitting position you can then switch to lay supine (face up–belly up) on the floor with your legs straight out and arms out to the sides. Relax and keep your attention on your teeth. This is the finish for Tooth Meditation and you can stay on the floor as long as you like.

Part Two

Once you become comfortable with Part One you can try Part Two:

Follow everything in Part One but reverse the position of your hands and legs so that the back of the hands are touching the chest with the pinky fingers pointing up to the nose and the thumbs dropped in the direction of the belly button, while the left ankle is crossed over the right knee to rest it there. The elbows are gently tugging backward.

Remember in Part One the fingers are resting on your breastbone? Now you imagine in your mind that the palms of your interlocked hands are behind your back and pressing gently against your spine. The mind plays the key role in Part Two.

Advanced Tooth Meditation

In addition to the Basic routine described above you can add another step for an advanced more active meditation.

Remember the "feeling" of chewing a thick piece of bubble gum. During the meditation imagine you are chewing gum and try to recreate all the feelings in the teeth, tongue, jaw muscles, and brain pleasure centers. But the piece of gum will be very very tiny while your tongue, teeth, and jaw muscles will be working in nano-micro-actions. The tongue stays touching the roof of the mouth and the top/bottom teeth stay barely touching. Everything should be moving in such a tiny scale that you would need a microscope to see.

The important gem in this advanced meditation is to discover the actual feel of the gum between your teeth. The feeling is your chi or energy.

This chapter should help you get a feel for how much your teeth should relax and touch during later discussions on active Tooth Meditation With High Intensity Interval Training session.

CHAPTER 10
TOOTH MEDITATION TO
FIGHT HEART DISEASE WITH
TEN TOES AND TWO TONGUES

You're doing everything your doctor recommends to prevent and fight heart disease and then your dentist tells you that harmful microorganisms can easily and quickly enter your bloodstream throughout the sheer number of highly permeable capillaries under the tongue which increases the likelihood of heart disease and stroke. Now what?

Dentists will advise you to control these bad microorganisms by keeping your mouth bacterial colonies in a healthy balance. You can do this by chewing and swishing thoroughly, around the teeth/gums and under the tongue, healthy bacteria found in fermented foods including vegetable, fruit, milk, seed, cereal grain and laboratory made supplements. It's also very important to clean your oral cavity by daily toothbrushing, flossing, tongue scraping and using herbal antimicrobial rinses.

If you are searching for more alternative ways to improve and maintain heart health I would like to introduce you to one of my favorite fun and easy to do heart healthy meditations. And all it takes is a tap of a foot and a lick of the tongue!

Did you know that every human has two hearts and two tongues? Yes, it's true...sort of! It's easy to feel the primary blood pumping heart muscle behind your rib cage sternum which beats about 100,000 times a day. You also have a "second heart" which is a system of muscles, veins, and valves deep in the calf and foot which pump deoxygenated blood back up to the heart and lungs.

Your second heart system, however, must actively contract/relax the surrounding leg muscles to pump the blood upward against gravity.

The best exercise to work the foot/leg muscle pump system and force blood back up to the chest cavity is simple walking. But many of us work 8 hour day jobs standing or sitting and then spend another 2-4 hours after work with more sitting in front of a television or home computer. This sedentary lifestyle doesn't allow time for the constant leg muscle stimulation required to properly move the approximate 2000 gallons of blood flowing through your network of blood vessels throughout the day. I'll show you the solution to this problem in a minute but first I want you to know more about your two tongues.

My book "Teeth In Mortal Combat" clearly relates the ancient Oriental theory about the tongue being an energetic extension of the heart. If you haven't read my book you might find this more believable if you accept the fact that many heart diseases are actually emotional in nature and it's easy to see how the tongue is a vital emotional outlet. If you are still skeptical then try practicing the following meditation for a month and feel the convincing results. You'll be pleasantly surprised when you discover your tongue-heart connection. (*http://www.amazon.com/s/ref=ntt_athr_dp_sr_1?_encoding=UTF8&sort=relevancerank&search-alias=books&field-author=Lester%20Sawicki%20DDS*)

Since the human body has two heart systems then according to ancient chi meridian energy principles it's only natural the tongue energy will extend through both hearts. Once your tongue energy passes through the chest heart it's energy extension will divide into two parts in order to pass through the heart system of both right and left legs. You'll see how this happens during the meditation. By the way, this is an excellent exercise that keeps your lower extremity blood flowing to prevent DVT deep vein thrombosis (blood clots in the legs) while suffering through the agony of sitting in the cramped seat of an airliner.

Here are the steps to help you become a tooth meditator:

Sit comfortably in a chair and relax all your muscles head to toe. Let your lips stay closed while breathing in and out through your nose. The teeth should touch together very lightly while the tip of the the tongue gently relaxes against the roof of the mouth. Swallow your saliva and then use your imagination to see and feel and curl the tip of the tongue inward/backward and stretching down the throat toward the chest heart. Use more of your imagination to direct the visualized tongue energy to wrap itself around your heart. Then imagine your energy into a self-massage and lick your heart with loving thoughts. Be aware of the pleasurable feelings that arise as your heart relaxes, softens and expands. Make just the slightest effort to smile and replace your heart with a picture of yourself as a happy baby and feel yourself being tickled on your tummy. Enjoy!

Once you have mastered massaging your heart use even more imagination to extend the tongue energy further down into the abdomen and split it into two so that each tongue continues to pass through the center of both legs to the tips of the toes. Keep the extended tongue feeling in mind as you begin tapping your foot-heel against the floor. Begin alternately tapping the balls of the feet and the heels firmly with any pattern and rhythm you like. You should stay relaxed and tap the heels firmly enough so that the vibration created travels through the leg bones and up the spine to the jaw bone and teeth. You should feel the slightest vibration running through your teeth and the surrounding jaw bone. Remember to completely relax the jaw and facial muscles and keep the teeth just barely touching together.

From time to time stop the tapping and keep the feet flat on the floor. Gently shake the legs in and out as if shivering. Keep your attention inside your body searching for any unusual feelings such as pressure, tingling or warmth. Repeat the foot tapping and then shake/shiver again. After a while still the entire body/mind system and focus on your breathing and heart beat. Try to relax and slow your breath by counting each inhale/exhale. Examine the way you feel in this relaxed state.

This sitting meditation creates a detoxifying whole body vibration not only through the bones but also the soft tissue of the body. Foot-heel tapping activates the second heart system with your calf and foot muscles pumping deoxygenated blood back up to the lungs and primary heart muscle. Shaking/shivering the legs stimulates the vagus (tenth cranial nerve) nerve endings in the pelvic area which activates the parasympathetic relaxation response. Visualizing and feeling tongue energy stimulates various energetic meridians throughout the body that help your chi flow more smoothly and uninterrupted. All these factors help improve physical and emotional health.

Sitting in a chair foot tapping and leg shaking for heart health is simple to do at any time of the day. It's perfect if you're a passenger in a car, taxi, bus, train, airplane, while watching a movie or play, and even better at a rock concert. It will awaken you into a positive frame of mind and keep you more alert. You can save the more relaxing tongue massage visualization for special quiet times of the day when you feel a real need to chill out.

For more information visit the Teeth Sensei at: *http://www.tooth-fight.com*

CHAPTER 11
TOOTH MEDITATION TURNS ON YOUR RELAXATION RESPONSE

Connect your mind with meditation and some physical action and you'll be able to switch on a <u>relaxation response</u>. The relaxation response is a parasympathetic state of body and mind that arises through the stimulation of the <u>Vagus (tenth cranial)</u> <u>nerve</u> which leads to positive body changes such as:

> slower heart rate
> lower blood pressure
> greater immunity
> overcoming inflammation
> less stress
> release of stem cells for tissue repair

According to Chinese Medicine theory the heart and lung are located in the area of the chest called the upper energizer. The heart governs blood and the lung governs qi. The circulation of heart blood depends on the help of lung qi moving it to ensure smooth circulation. Deficient heart qi can affect the health of the lungs leading to congestion. If you want healthy lungs the heart has to be pumping efficiently and for a strong heart the lungs have to breathe fully and clearly. For more information on Chinese medicine visit <u>Jade Spirit Community Acupuncture</u>.

This explains why aerobic exercise benefits both heart and lungs and a cardiac pacemaker helps prevent fluid accumulation in the lungs. The vagus is involved in the efficient functioning of the lungs and its stimulation is a key stage in relaxation meditation.

It can be stimulated in many ways one of which is pressing the tongue against the palate and swallowing your saliva.

The vagus nerve contributes to tongue movement through the palatoglossus muscle. Some dental patients have trouble relaxing their tongue during dental procedures. It fidgets, darts and pushes with extreme forces against any dental instrument it comes into contact with. The thrusting and side to side tongue lashing is one of dentistry's greatest frustrations and limitations to quality treatment. That's why every dentist is trained and tested in the exceptional martial arts of tongue fighting. You can be sure that your dentist has earned a black belt in the specialized fighting art of the "way of no tongue."–:)

In jest, the tongue is such a formidable opponent that we often have no choice but to resort to the "dim mak" touch of death with a shot of novocaine temporarily numbing it with partial paralysis obedient to our every command. And now you know how the legendary TV kung fu artist "Caine" was named. :)

Actually, if you have read *Teeth In Mortal Combat* you'll understand why your tongue is your best friend and should be treated with the highest respect it deserves. The following meditation will help you become more familiar with your tongue and it's natural ability to support strong healthy heart and lungs.

Here's the drill:

Sit straight up and relaxed in a chair with feet resting flat against the floor. To relax and set your focus warm up with these two exercises that help prevent wrinkles. Smile wide, try to wiggle your ears and then pucker-kiss your lips hard. Repeat several times. Then without causing pain pinch and jiggle all the loose skin on your face for a second such as:

>   between the eyebrows at the nose bridge
>   the eyebrows

temple

below the ears at the edge of the jawbone

along the jawbone

lower middle upper cheeks near the jawbone

upper middle lower cheeks near the nose

Now we begin the tooth meditation:

1.) Inhale and exhale deeply and completely in a relaxed manner through your nose during the entire exercise. When you begin the inhale you should feel your stomach relax and stretch out a little just as if you were laying supine on the floor. At the point of fully inhaled lungs you should notice the slightest tension in your shoulders as they barely pull back and the ribs expand outward and forward. Never force your breathing. After some experience with this type of abdomen breathing you can progress to more <u>advanced diaphragmatic breathing</u>.

2.) Open your mouth wide, stick out your tongue and grab it firmly between thumb and forefinger using a small dry 2x2 gauze, cut cloth or paper towel. Relax your tongue and allow it to retract slightly back into your mouth. Close your eyes and relax the eyelids, neck, jaw, lips and facial muscles.

3.) Begin by gently pulling and shaking, side-to-side, your relaxed tongue with a firm finger grip. Be careful to avoid injuring the frenum muscle attachment located under the tongue. Don't pull too hard and avoid rubbing the frenum against the incisal edges of the lower front teeth. Shake the tongue from side to side for 60 seconds then pull it in and out for about 30 seconds and finally end the exercise by rotating it in a circular direction for a while. You can repeat this again if you aren't tired and secreted saliva isn't overflowing your lips.

4.) When you are finished place your hands on your thighs and relax for a few moments paying special attention to your heart and breath. Focus on any unusual feelings you are experiencing in the area between the inner spine and sternum plus the diamond space between the bridge of the nose, ears and cervical vertebrae. Smile!

This meditation should have far reaching positive effects. According to Chinese medicine the heart and lung organs are reflected to the tip of the tongue. My theory is that with acupressure pinching the area you are stimulating the energy flow to the two organs. Pulling and shaking the tongue activates the vagus nerve through the palatoglossus muscle. The end result is encouraging the body to shift into a parasympathetic relaxation response.

For more information visit the Teeth Sensei at: *www.toothfight.com*

Chapter 12
TOOTH MEDITATION TO MAXIMIZE HIGH INTENSITY INTERVAL TRAINING FOR LONGEVITY

If longevity is one of your goals then Tooth Meditation might be for you. It all begins with a simple question: Do you believe that searching for enlightenment is like climbing a mountain?

If you want to be enlightened on your quest for longevity then you had better pick your mountain carefully. The extreme exercise and process of climbing Mt. Everest to it's peek or its opposite competitive free-diving into the deep sea might enlighten you but it can also kill you or at least reduce your life expectancy if attempted too many times.

For longevity, I wouldn't spend too much time at the extreme intensity side of living. A rule of thumb is if you can't have and enjoy safe sex at your point in time then you could be cutting short your lifespan. Having sex to propagate the human race is hard-wired into our DNA and anything that interferes with this function will likely reduce your lifespan if not bring us to extinction.

Humans don't have sex in trees because it's too dangerous. Your family tree would be pretty short if your great grandparents had spent much time on a limb and you might never had been born. If you're in a safe environment and can adjust your mind to relax into love then the space is ripe to promote longevity. Extreme intense exercise isn't the right space for longevity and if repeated on a regular basis your lifespan will probably suffer.

You get the drift…which is why I recommend incorporating periodic sessions of Tooth Meditation into your fitness workouts.

My understanding is that fitness scientists are more interested in researching extreme intense competitive performance based exercise rather than exercise for longevity because that's where the money is. Who wouldn't want to perform at a higher level to win in today's competitive environment? That's why I decided to ignore some of what is being promoted as today's best exercise for longevity. Too much of it seems fixated on competition and winning, as if you can accumulate enough points to win 120 years.

When you exercise for longevity ask yourself, "am I spending too much time balancing on a tree limb trying to improve my performance and one-up a win against my fellow athletes or am I really exercising for longevity?" Consider Tooth Meditation and apply it to your fitness routine for a more reasonable approach to exercise for a longer healthy life. My mantra is it's ok to occasionally "visit" the peek and depth of earth's wonders but a longer life comes from regular smarter exercise.

Pick up any current book or magazine that features fitness advice and you'll certainly read about "HIIT" high intensity interval training.

http://www.hussmanfitness.org/html/TGHowtoWorkout.html
http://en.wikipedia.org/wiki/High-intensity_interval_training
Since the late 1990's clinical studies of well conditioned athletes showed that HIIT is the most effective type of cardiovascular exercise that improves performance, especially when one can't overcome a plateau in training. "Wind sprints" are the most common exercise used with high intensity interval training.

Personal trainers today are recommending HIIT for the general public as a tool for fat burning and achieving higher levels of fitness. And although the HIIT regimen is proven to improve performance for many athletes as well as the casual fitness enthusiast, it has not been proven to increase longevity or maintain health. More research has to be done here.

Unless you are a competitive athlete trying to improve performance you might want to give more thought to the intensity of your sprints. What level of exertion would give best results for longevity? And if you believe in "no pain no gain" with maximum intensity then it might be that, according to Cialdini, you could be having a difficult time changing your old belief system because humans have a built in tendency to keep thoughts and beliefs consistent with what has already been done or decided. (*http://www.managementconsultingnews.com/interviews/cialdini_interview.php*)

As an example, I haven't been a competitive athlete since high school and it's taken me over 40 years to overcome my questionable belief system that extremely hard exercise benefits me. That's why I'm concerned that people in general may fall into the same trap I did of taking HIIT into the realm of extreme exercise rather than adapt it for longevity. (*http://medicalxpress.com/news/2011-08-lifestyles-healthy-defy.html*)

Most of my research points to the fact that today's high tech generation would benefit more by incorporating a slightly higher value of parasympathetic over sympathetic nervous system activity when health maintenance and longevity is the goal. Parasympathetic state includes "rest and digest" and is the main function engaged during recovery and meditation. Much of humanity today is stressed out and lacking enough parasympathetic activity to stay in homeostatic relaxed balance. That's why I'm suggesting a sprinkle of parasympathetic spice into your wind sprint high intensity interval training. (*http://en.wikipedia.org/wiki/ Parasympathetic_nervous_system*)

The easiest triggers for parasympathetic stimulation is intended relaxation and swallowing saliva. The vagus nerve (tenth cranial nerve) is one of the most important parasympathetic nerves originating in the brain and it travels to all the major organs. It has a connection with the tongue and is a key player in the swallow/ gag reflex. When you intentionally swallow the vagus is activated which in turn switches on a signal that stimulates the entire relax-digest system network in the body. If you're interested in longevity then relaxation and satisfaction with life should become a natural part of your existence.

It's been scientifically shown that the vagus nerve:

Reduces inflammation

Activates stem cells that help regenerate organs

Increases heart function

Boosts immunity

Reduces stress

Here's the drill:

Parasympathetic activity mixed into your high intensity interval training wind sprints requires you to stay relaxed and loose during and after the sprint and to <u>not</u> strive for extreme exertion. Personal experience has shown me that staying relaxed is not an easy physical and emotional state to maintain while sprinting "just hard enough."

Keep these keys in mind during and after sprinting:
1. Relax the facial muscle including lips.
2. Relax the arms and especially hands.
3. The tip of tongue to be relaxed against palate.
4. Top and bottom teeth gently touching together.

5. Lips closed, if possible, and breathe thru nose.
6. When sprinting feel the teeth vibrate lightly against each other.
7. Keep your attention on the soles of your feet hitting the sprinting surface.
8. Swallow your saliva at the top of your inhale and bottom of exhale.
9. Imagine the saliva traveling all the way to the bottom of your feet.

The above list, plus more, is what you might encounter if you entered a meditation class. For those of you without any experience in meditation I've reduced the nine keys to the simplest combination:

1. Relax and swallow your saliva after each inhale and exhale.
2. Chill out and do the best you can without slipping into extreme exertion.

Accumulating enough saliva to swallow is more difficult than relaxing. Salivary production is related with what you had to eat and drink the day of and before, nutritional supplements and herbs you take, the drugs you are on, your hormonal balance, ambient temperature and humidity, how well you can relax and the degree of physical exhaustion.

You likely won't be able to swallow as often when you tire. However, at no time should you ever place a candy or gum in your mouth to help stimulate saliva production. The danger of aspirating into the lung is too great! Just relax and swallow whenever you can.

You can create more saliva naturally by relaxing, opening the mouth wide, smiling, sucking on your tongue, smacking your lips with your tongue, and other oral maneuvers which you'll naturally discover. If you can't swallow then just relax and feel the top and bottom teeth lightly touching against each other. Don't clench!

What's important is your decision to do HIIT for longevity and not for increased performance. Don't sprint into extreme exhaustion. It's normal that your body will tense as you tire but the idea is to use your mind to stay as relaxed as possible. Activate the "relax and digest" parasympathetic nervous system during the session. You should feel positive about the training and if you start to slip into a negative attitude just relax, smile, and see the smiling baby in your lower abdomen, a common meditative visualization that supports healthy "feel good" emotions. (*http://www.universal-tao.com/article/the_inner_smile.html*)

Chapter 13
MENTAL SOCCER TURNS ON LONGEVITY GENES WITH HIIT

First, let's remember that there are no cases cited, in my research, where centenarians either worked, played or exercised to extreme limits with regularity. And with that in mind one has to decided on the purpose of one's exercise and assemble it's workings logically. What I'm discussing is exercise for longevity and not performance.

It's been scientifically documented that regular sessions of extreme exercise will stimulate your body to release "feel good" endorphins, such as when a marathon runner experiences a runner's high. But endorphins are also released in long term meditators by just sitting, resting and watching which is one of the physiological benefits of meditation. (*http://www.telegraph.co.uk/health/dietandfitness/3321984/How-to-hit-a-natural-high.html*)

So think twice when you read about studies which favor the benefits of high intensity interval training. None of them can document examples of longevity for humans. Common sense would caution one to follow a more moderate path as we have witnessed with past and living centenarians.

The key to a vibrant workout is "feeling" vibrations. The very first suggestion to help you feel vibrations is to either walk and sprint barefoot or wear shoes constructed with ultrathin soles such as slippers, moccasins and barefoot running shoes. I currently wear Vibram Five Fingers and because of their growing popularity competing shoe manufacturers are designing new minimalist entries which are jumping onto store shelves. (*http://www.barefootrunner.com/*)

Today most athletic shoes have shock absorbing soles designed to stop vibration from traveling foot to spine which manufacturers claim prevent hip and knee stress injuries. This type of shoe is counterproductive to tooth meditation. Creating and feeling shock vibrations requires a bare foot or thin soled foot covering to bring your step into a mini shock against a hard surface.

Secondly, for your body (especially teeth) to vibrate effectively you have to find the right balance in your structural posture between too relaxed or too pumped up. Think of your body as a soccer ball or guitar string. You have to find the right pressure and tension that allows best performance. It's surprisingly easy and you'll have good results if you don't over think it.

There's lots of fun you can have feeling the energetic effects of tooth meditation with HIIT.

1. As you recover with walking between sprints imagine and feel as if you are stepping on and crushing a soda can. If you have trouble feeling this try walking with your big toe lifted up.

With every step crushing the can imagine and feel biting into hard chewing gum. The visualized gum should be pretty resistant to deformation so you can concretely feel it with your jaw muscles and between your teeth. (CAUTION: Never ever chew gum or have any kind of food or snack in your mouth while exercising with HIIT.) Remember that the teeth never clench but just lightly touch, if at all. The tongue should be pressing against the roof of the mouth.

If you continue having trouble imagining and feeling vibrations and/or chewing gum between your teeth then I suggest you investigate personal instruction in teeth qigong classes by *www. Fit-150.com.*

2. Longevity exercise should be effective and playful. Extreme effort without feeling like a child is not playful. Kids laugh and play with short bursts of energy. That's how I visualize myself during high intensity interval training.

Playing soccer is a childhood experience that is strongly embedded in my memory so when I run my sprints I imagine running after a soccer ball with a short burst of energy. When I reach the ball I slow down a micro tad in order to dribble it then immediately push it ahead with my mind so I can explode towards it again. I repeat this playful acting over and over.

> Push the ball forward with my mind
> Burst of energy to catch up to it
> Slow a tad to dribble
> Push it forward with my mind
> Explode to catch it
> Slow to dribble, etc.

3. According to a study from Virginia Tech, being able to see progress toward your goal will help you reach it. (*http://www. sciencedaily.com/releases/2011/08/110815143935.htm*)

This theory fits well with my soccer ball visualization as I can see my progress sprinting after the ball, reaching it and then pushing it forward to catch it again, which helps me finish the sprint with gusto. It also makes my HIIT session more playful, positive and satisfying as I never fail to catch up to the ball.

Chapter 14
ADVANCED TOOTH MEDITATION WITH HIIT

Introduction

Let me remind you of my strong feeling that the parasympathetic nervous system should be activated during longevity exercise with HIIT. Remember this training is intense and to adjust it for longevity you have to temper it with mental work. At various times during the training session your teeth should be lightly touching, the tip of the tongue touches your roof of mouth behind the upper front teeth and you're breathing through the nose. You'll know your on the right track if you can feel your cheeks relax into a jello-jiggle during the brief times of parasympathetic activation.

You can incorporate more mental work into your training by focusing on your thumbs. The opposable thumb has helped the human species develop more accurate fine motor skills and, according the Chinese Meridian theory, the fine motor skills of the hand directly enhance brain function. Follow these tips to enhance fitness, brain power, and longevity.

The exterior tip of the thumb is the endpoint for the lung meridian which runs on the inside of the arm beginning at the third intercostal space. The Lung meridian is the "Master of Respiration", therefore its acupuncture points are used for health of the lung, respiratory system and heart.

The lung meridian also represents the oxygen content of the body. It controls the exterior of the body and all the Yin-Meridians. It's reactions are most sensitive to harmful external influences (such as wind). Discords of the lung normally relate to a lack of Yin.

The Lung meridian has a close relationship with the meridians of the heart and circulatory system. It runs through the diaphragm and connects with the Large Intestines in the abdomen. A disturbance in the lungs can cause a disturbance in the abdomen (in Stomach, Liver, Gallbladder, Bladder, Pancreas) and in the pelvis area (Intestines, Kidneys, Prostate) and vice versa.

According to Ayurvedic Theory the hands have a power of their own which can help a person control his life. There is a tremendous flow of energy in our hands and each finger represents one of the five elements—the thumb is agni (fire), the forefinger is vayu (air), the middle finger is akash (ether), the ring finger is prithvi (earth) and the little finger is jal (water). The roots of all diseases lie in an imbalance of one of the five elements and can be corrected with herbal medicines, will power and Mudras.

In Western Medicine the lungs and heart are the two prime indicators of health and longevity. Studies have shown that the easiest way to predict a person's lifespan is to test lung function. Increase your lung function and you'll live longer. Focus on your thumbs during HIIT and the energy flow to the lungs and heart will move toward balance hopefully increasing your lifespan.

Technique Breathing Through Nose And Thumbs

During your HIIT remember all the suggestion from my past posts. When you activate your parasympathetic phase during the training session breathe through your nose and relax your nose, ears, neck, shoulders, arms, thumbs and forefingers. Imagine there is a flexible straw running from your thumbs up through your arm-shoulder-neck-ears and to your nose and inhale through your thumbs all the way to your nose. Exhale out your forefingers.

In a way you are breathing through your arm and hand. This sends energy through the thumb-forefinger—lung-heart circuit which will help activate your energy body into a longevity response.

Post Training Recovery

Much later in the day when you're taking a comfortable walk you can practice some gentle abdominal breathing with Tooth Meditation. This type of breath work is baffling for many beginning meditators. Actually, abdominal breathing is the normal physiologic state of the body when taking a relaxing walk, sitting, or lying on your back. The problem is living in today's stressful world has helped us forget how to breathe naturally in a healthful way. Under stress we tend to breathe more upper body with the lungs and chest.

Follow all the prior posts on *Tooth Meditation While Walking* and add this to them:

Walk backwards during this exercise.

Rest the palms of both your hands behind your back on your hips with the heels of the hand pressing gently "under" the ribcage at the location of the kidneys.

As you inhale, press a little more firmly on the kidneys with the heel of both hands and slightly tense up your back muscles to resist, plus, slightly tense your lower abdominal muscles all the way to the pubic bone. You will gently push out the lower abdomen and pretend to fill it with air from the inhale. (Physiologically you can't fill the lower abdomen with air but what happens is that the mind concentrates your chi to this area which is an important concept in Chinese meditation.) Continue into a full inhale as you fill up your lungs completely to your neck.

As you exhale, relax the hand pressure on your kidneys and relax the abdomen muscles and then repeat the first three steps with the next inhale. Be sure to relax everything with each exhale.

Whenever you feel like the time is right, turn around and walk forward for a while. Then switch around and walk backward again. Don't stress and tire yourself as this is for relaxation and recovery.

For more information on tooth meditation exercise visit the Teeth Sensei at: *www.tooth-fight.com*

60

Chapter 15
TOOTH MEDITATION BREATHING
WITH YOUR EARS

Your Eustachian tube, a 35 mm long tube that connects the pharynx to the middle ear, is normally closed. When diving even a few feet in water, climbing high up a mountain, or flying in an aircraft the difference in atmospheric pressure can create pain. Our Eustachian tube can open to let a small amount of air through to prevent damage by equalizing pressure between the middle ear and the atmosphere. Swallowing, yawning, chewing gum, or performing a valsava maneuver may be used intentionally to open the tube and equalize atmospheric pressure.

Science doesn't know exactly why people yawn. Some believe yawning gets more oxygen into the lungs and brain, while others say it helps cool the brain. Psychotherapists say that yawning is a way for the nervous system to discharge energy and teachers of meditation claim that yawning releases negative energy.

Physiologically, yawning:

is initiated by the parasympathetic nervous system
boosts your blood pressure
increases your heart rate
stretches the ear drum

Considering all the above, you could say yawning arouses the person into a more alert state, perfect for active meditation.

Many teachers of meditation give instruction on whole body breathing. One of the claimed benefits is cleansing your internal chi by exchanging the dirty energy inside your body with surrounding pure energy of nature. Another purpose is to take outside energy and pack it internally to make your chi more dense and available for healing or self-defense.

Whole body breathing is a concept difficult for novice meditators to grasp and, to make it easier, teachers will often break it down into smaller sections such as breathing with the skin of the hands, feet, bones, organs, blood vessels, nose, and eyes etc.

I recommend breathing with the ears to initiate and simulate whole body breathing during tooth meditation. Results are quick and you'll easily feel more centered, balanced, harmonized, and in the zone for deep meditation.

It's a little tricky at first, but to get yourself into the right state for ear breathing you begin with an open mouth yawn. As you hold your yawn, you'll feel your ear drums stretch and Eustachian tubes open. Keep the mouth open, close your throat, and begin breathing through the nose only while you continue to yawn. Now close your mouth and continue breathing through your nose and ears, with ear drums stretched and open Eustachian tubes. Focus on your ears and feel the slight change of pressure in your ears. Once you get this feeling you keep it and imagine you are breathing in and out your ears.

Here are the physical signs that you are in the right mode for ear breathing:

1.   You experience "autophony", the hearing of self-generated sounds. These sounds, such as one's own breathing, voice, and heartbeat, vibrate directly onto the ear drum and can create a "bucket on the head" effect or muffled "water in the ear" hearing.

2.   Your trachea has more volume when the Eustachian tube is open and your voice may sound lower to other people.

3.   If you hum a sound, such as "ohm", the increased volume you hear with greater vibration will make you think your teeth might jump right out of their bony sockets. Your skull and brainstem

will vibrate at an intensity you've never thought possible. You'll feel like a Tibetan Monk chanting in deep meditation, centered and peaceful.

4. As you force air out your nose during aerobic exercise, you'll feel pressure push out your eardrums.

You can practice ear breathing in sitting or walking meditation, even during High Intensity Interval Training.

Links related to this article:

http://en.wikipedia.org/wiki/Eustachian_tube

http://www.prevention.com/health/fitness/tips-for-success/a-yawning-problem/article/9c69d08f88803110VgnVCM20000012281eac_____

http://www.sciencebase.com/science-blog/yawning-cools-the-brain.html

http://en.wikipedia.org/wiki/Yawn

http://www.ncbi.nlm.nih.gov/pubmed/8902321

http://www.myshrink.com/counseling-theory.php?t_id=82

http://baillement.com/english/yawn-triggered.html

Yawn Of A Tortoise

http://blogs.scientificamerican.com/scicurious-brain/2011/10/01/ignobel-prize-winner-if-you-yawn-your-pet-tortoise-dont-care/

http://www.youtube.com/watch?feature=player_embedded&v=zvyHhdaEA-k

CHAPTER 16
TRAP-JAW DANCING MEDITATION

"Odontomachus, commonly called trap-jaw ant, is a genus of carnivorous ants found in the tropics and subtropics throughout the world. According to Wikipedia, they have a large, straight mandible capable of opening 180 degrees. The mandibles have the fastest moving predatory appendages in the animal kingdom. They are powerful and fast and can snap shut on prey to kill or maim, but they also permit slow and fine movements. They can also capture and catapult away an intruder as well as fling themselves backward to escape a threat." (*http://en.wikipedia.org/wiki/ Odontomachus*)

Now I ask you to see if the YouTube video is still playing, "Yoga demonstrated by a Tibetan Yogi" (*http://www.youtube. com/watch?v=APttKuYgwUA*) or you can see the video on my website at: *http://teethfight.com/index.php?page=videos_articles& logout=1&list2=1.* Carefully watch the action of the upper arm slapping against the armpit and ribcage. This is a good view of a trap-jaw arm slowly open and explode shut. After reading this chapter you'll be able to incorporate in your life the energetic aspect of a trap-jaw.

The dance of life, meditation dance, martial arts dance, kung fu dance, tai chi dance. All dance is an expression of energy and if you want to develop power in your dance you've got to engage the enormous potential energy in your jaws and teeth. I've named the exercise of this energy as "trap-jaw dancing."

Most people don't think about the reservoir of energy in their jaws and its power to expand human potential. The masseter jaw muscle is often considered the strongest muscle in the body. Your teeth are the hardest and longest living substance in your body. Even after death, a tooth with its crystal structure is a treasure holding the memory of your life and can survive millions of years buried in the earth.

In addition, did you know that the most basic instinct for survival is found in your teeth and jaws? Masters of martial arts don't teach this secret for the same reason the development and strengthening of teeth/jaws has been repressed by society. In my opinion, the reason is inherent control issues involved with honoring and cultivating this particular instinct. You can read all about the tragic cover-up in my book, *Teeth In Mortal Combat, How to Unleash Your Most Basic Instinct for Survival.*

Trap-jaw dancing is active meditation using mental weight training that you can integrate into all aspects of your life. During the exercise your mind should tire, but not to exhaustion, and with practice you'll experience the pleasurable slow, juicy feeling of endorphins flowing through your system. It is advisable to first get familiar with the energetic feeling of chewing an imaginary thick, resistant, sticky clump of bubblegum before you try trap-jaw dancing.

These are the basic preparation steps:

a.) Put your mind in a relaxed state and stand comfortably with arms at your side.

b.) Bend your elbows outward enough to open the space in your armpit so that you clearly feel the air in your armpit and the bicep is not touching the ribs.

c.) Imagine an inflatable ball smaller than a volleyball, deep in your armpit, trapped between your upper arm and ribcage, your upper arm holding it in place against a ribcage that expands outward a little.

d.) Your imaginary ball changes in size as your arm moves in any direction, straight up 180 degrees, outward 90 degrees, or down. Remember, the armpit space never collapses to the point where the arm touches the ribs. The imaginary ball is always in place.

Use your mind and magnetic energy that radiates from your body to suck up the ball into your armpit space. Imagine the feeling of holding a ball in your armpit that expands and shrinks as you arm moves in different directions and don't let it drop from your armpit. Always hold it in your armpit no matter the size it becomes. You should look and feel like the "Michelin Tire" man.

Once you get the feel, you can slowly walk with the imaginary ball in your armpit, or jog, sprint, dance, and practice your martial art. I enjoy feeling the ball as I drive my car with hands on the steering wheel. Consistent practice triggers endorphins which will give you a relaxed, focused and alert, stimulating buzz.

Trap-Jaw Meditation

Now you're ready to try the trap-jaw meditation, especially if you're getting good results with the bubblegum feeling. You should imagine a thick sticky clump in your mouth which has strong resistance to biting and sticks to your teeth making it hard to pull your teeth apart.

1.) Imagine, see and feel your head and neck including seven cervical vertebra in each shoulder. Your top teeth are in your upper arm and the lower teeth in your ribcage. The shoulder joint is your temporal mandibular joint (TMJ).

2.) See the imaginary ball in your armpits and imagine that you are biting into it. The ball has bubblegum-like properties and sticks to your teeth as your jaw opens to pull the ball apart and make it larger; again, squeeze the ball with your teeth.

3.) Your mind keeps it sucked into your armpit/imaginary jaw. Feel the ball with your teeth and squeeze into it. Pull it apart as your jaw/armpit opens, even to 180 degrees. The jaws and arm work together holding the ball in place, squeezing and stretching it apart as it resists in both directions.

4.) You'll know you understand this if you feel your jaws, ears and neck muscles tense a little.

With practice, you'll experience your teeth tingle as they fill with energy. Your jaws will get a puffed up feeling. Your head will screw on straighter as the seven cervical vertebra readjust into better alignment. With consistent practice you'll eventually be able to explode your arm as shown in the Tibetan Yoga video.

Yes, your oral cavity has poetic passion and I hope this chapter gave you a glimpse of how the teeth and jaws can be used to screw your head on straighter for a more connected, flowing, and powerful energetic dance.

Chapter 17
TOOTH RUBBING MEDITATION FOR INCREASED BRAIN POWER

The human brain is considered one of the most complex organic entities in the known universe and there are many myths about it and how it works. One myth is that people use only 10% of their brains and a person may harness the unused potential to increase intelligence. Factors of intelligence can increase with training, but technological leaps in brain scanning has proved this 10% rule to be false and even doing something simple, such as clenching your fist, uses much more than 10% of the brain. Cognitive enhancing drugs, however, such as modafinil, normally prescribed for sleep disorders, and Ritalin and Adderall, taken for ADHD, can help us increase memory and focus.

Many spiritual New Age theories peddle the belief that the dormant 90% of our brain is capable of exhibiting psychic powers and can be trained to perform psychokinesis and extra-sensory perception. I believe that some people are born with psychic ability, but there is no scientifically verified body of evidence supporting the idea that such powers can be taught to the average person.

What I find really interesting is that, in terms of oxygen and nutrient consumption, the brain can require up to twenty percent of the body's energy—more than any other organ—despite equalling only 2% of the human body weight. Common sense tells me that you can increase your brain "power" with exercise, both physical and mental. Your brain is like a muscle, the more you use it the stronger and sharper it becomes.

Ancient teachings about boosting brain power through mastering the 5 Excellencies of painting, poetry, calligraphy, medicine and martial arts are now supported with scientific studies. And there are many simple exercises that can help you stay brain fit without spending both years and a small fortune studying complicated Eastern Arts.

Brain exercises using mindfulness meditation programs are growing in popularity because they are easy to learn, with minimal investment of money, and appear to make measurable changes in brain regions associated with memory, sense of self, empathy, and stress. The common problem with some meditations, however, is the tendency for beginners to fall asleep as they become more and more relaxed.

This won't happen with tooth meditation which engages the mind with active physical movement. If you fall asleep during tooth meditation, then you are either too tired to be practicing this form of meditation, or your body suffers a sleep deficit. Both instances should be addressed and corrected before delving into this meditative exercise.

Tooth Rubbing Meditation engages the 3 senses of touch, sight, and hearing. Sight involves imagining and seeing, with your inner eye, your tooth glowing bright like a lantern in the dark. Your sense of touch will be activated by the movement of your index fingertip rubbing against the enamel of your tooth. As you rub your tooth you'll hear a squeaky sound similar to running your finger around the lip of a crystal glass bowl.

Three reasons to engage your senses are:

A.) Using your imagination to see your tooth light up gives you a reference point in inner space in addition to the outer space of gravity pulling on the bottom of your feet, if you're stand-ing, or pelvis if you're sitting. This helps give better balance to the body while integrating the right and left hemispheres of the brain.

B.) It's been proven that engaging the fingers to perform tasks can increase brain power. The nerve endings in the fingers lead directly to your brain and moving them increases brain cir-culation. Studies that have mapped the brain show the tips of the fingers correspond to more areas located in the brain than any other part of the body. Exercising them actually enlarge the brain's capacity and increase the number of connections between neurons creating new neural pathways.

C.) You'll boost your brain power even further if you use your non-dominant hand to perform this simple meditation. Do-ing so will stimulate the flow of energy to the more neglected, opposite side of your brain.

Here are the 9 easy steps for Tooth Rubbing Meditation:

1.) It's important that your teeth and fingers are squeaky clean. You might want to brush your teeth for a few seconds with a dry toothbrush or use some natural toothpaste/powder.

2.) Put yourself into a relaxed state of mind and body, standing or sitting comfortably.

3.) Close the lips and lightly touch the upper and lower teeth while relaxing the jaw and facial muscles, including lips, cheeks, nose, eyes, and ears.

4.) Touch the top of your palate behind your front teeth with the tip of your tongue.

5.) Breathe through your nose, if possible.

6.) Swallow any saliva that accumulates. Visualize it as a round

sun and mentally follow it's transport to your lower abdomen. Use your imagination and pretend you can see and feel
your saliva as a bright warm sun glowing in the center of your
abdomen beneath the navel.

7.) Keep your arms relaxed at your sides if standing; or resting
on your lap, stomach, or chair while sitting. Make an effort to
relax the muscles in your fingers, hand, arm, shoulder, neck,
jaw.

8.) Relax and gently breathe each exhale into your finger joints,
wrist, elbow, shoulder, tmj, jaw bone and teeth all the way to
your chin. Pretend there's a flexible small diameter tube traveling through your throat connecting your nose to each bone
of these body parts.

9.) In your mind preset a timing interval for each stage of your
breathing. Many meditation instructors would give you a pre-
determined rhythm such as:

- *Slowly inhale for a count of 4 seconds.*
- *Hold your breath for 4 seconds.*
- *Slowly exhale, as you count in your mind, for 4–8 seconds.*
- *Hold your breath 2 seconds.*
- *Inhale again 4–6 seconds.*
- *Hold you breath 4 seconds.*
- *Slowly exhale as you count in your mind 8 seconds.*
- *Hold your breath 4 seconds.*
- *Repeat with a rhythm that feels comfortable.*

The rhythm is arbitrary. What's important is that, as a beginner,
you do not strain your breathing at any point in the cycle.

10) Once you have some meditation experience with a comfortable breathing/counting rhythm you take your non-dominant hand fingertip and begin rubbing the face side of an
upper front tooth creating friction until you hear a squeaking

sound. Rub up and down in a vertical direction. There's a trick to getting just the right rub for a squeak to sound. You might have to use your tongue to wet the tooth a little and play with moisture on the tooth to get the squeak.

Once your tooth starts singing, you squeak it in sync with every count during the breath work. You'll be amazed at how loud the sound is to your ears as the tooth vibrations echo via the bones, air spaces, and sinuses of your skull. Rest assured you won't fall asleep in this meditation, listening to the squeaks while your concentration focuses on all the little steps involved. The idea is to reach deeper levels of relaxation without falling asleep.

The final optional visualization uses your mind's eye to see the tooth light up, like a lantern, brighter and brighter with each rub.

The overall benefits of tooth rubbing meditation for increased brain power is profound.

Chapter 18
NOT A MASTER YET?...
THERE ARE REASONS

Do you see yourself as the typical martial arts student striving to go beyond just training your dragon; you want to "change" your dragon through meditation?

Sorry strivers, your dragon (the DNA you were born with) matters. Your success in life is determined 50% by your genes, 50% by your environment, and 100% by your desire. And if you vow to "chew bitters" in order to become as good or better than your master teacher, be ready to give 200% with an almost guarantee of failure because your genes, environment, and teacher will get in your way.

Your DNA predetermines what you can become and there's no proof, in either science, religion, magic, or spiritual teachings, that it's possible to change the genetics you were born with. And every person's dragon has a different talent which can be trained, but not changed. If you try to become just like your teacher, with all his mental/physical strength and paranormal abilities, you have a high possibility of failure no matter how many schools and techniques of meditation you pursue. Your teacher was born with special skills and his teacher, your grandmaster, recognized and helped him develop these skills beyond the normal person's ability and imagination.

Unfortunately, many teachers continue to toy with the ploy of "transmitting" secrets only to devotees of their lineage. Followers are distracted by the supernormal powers of their guru and hope to change their average ability, through years of hard physical work and meditation, into a replica of a guru that can perform paranormal feats such as break rocks with their mind, disarm an opponent with a stream of chi, control the weather, climb snowy mountains dressed in wet sheets, levitate, erase karma, and soak in the splendor of nirvana, etc.

It's time for you to realize that you are unique and should develop your own talents. Each person has a separate identity that can't be cloned and trying to clothe yourself with the mystique of your teacher is futile endeavor. A spiritual teacher shows you a path toward self-realization, not cookie-cutter cloning of his expert ability.

I hope after reading this chapter you'll have a clearer picture of reality. Now is the time to recognize you can train, but not change your dragon. Your teacher should help you discover and nurture your dragon to become all it can be. Don't make the mistake of trying to kidnap and clone your teacher's dragon.

But what, you may ask, does it mean to use your mind and energy to bring about personal transformation? Heating the cauldron to a boil? Tempering iron into an enlightenment sword of steel? Washing your bone marrow to create a pearl of heavenly wisdom and health? Transmutation of mercury into gold? Condensing your chi into a golden elixir of immortality?

After all, the water turns to steam, right? And the sword protects you with ... invincible power? How about the age old adage of repeating an exercise 100,000 times in order to "burn" it into your consciousness so you can muster the grand ultimate skill of mastery? Doesn't all the accumulated "psychic heat" create a real alchemical change in your chi and being?

Sorry, strivers: DNA and talent still matters. Yes, quality can and is always changing. It's the law of nature. But the nature of all things remains the same in our earthly dimension and there is no proof, only theories, of what is possible in "other dimensions" and how they operate.

So I am suggesting we stay real and focus on becoming all we can in our known universe, using the talents we are born with. Imagination can only take us to a point. Did you ever consider the millions of students of martial arts and meditation that never developed beyond the skill of an average person? Where's the proof that you can change your DNA? In a manner of speaking, almost all devotees striving for a spiritual banquet eventually come back to the meat on their kitchen table.

Let's get real…

… and review what science has discovered, so far, about people with supernormal abilities and the likelihood of teaching others their special skill:

If you expect to become a martial arts master you need to be mentally disciplined and focused with a combination and interaction of genetics, incredible and unique training, special and usually private experience with another master, and an obsessive drive to achieve and persevere.

Many super humans have an oversized heart that beats over 200 times a minute pumping an extraordinary large volume of blood and oxygen to the limbs. Their lungs can take in an extremely high amount of oxygen. Super fit people have muscle performance that is partly determined by muscle cell efficiency in using sugar as a fuel source. They have an abundance of specific protein receptors which can increase exercise capacity because the cells are better at taking up sugar from the blood stream, storing it, and burning it for energy. They are more efficient in complete mitochondrial burning of fuel. They can run faster and longer. Their muscles produce at least half as much lactic acid allowing much faster recovery than average people.

Scientists found that people had better endurance if they had inherited the so-called I allele of the angiotensin-converting enzyme (ACE) gene. The best performances were seen in people who had inherited the I allele from both parents. Other researchers discovered that having functional alpha-actinin-3 improves power performance in muscle and speed. In people of European descent, 18% have the alpha-actinin-3 deficient genotype. In Asians, the frequency is 25%.

Paranormal feats are always associated with specific brain synaptic discharges that are not seen in the usual day-to-day activity of normal people.

Myostatin-related Muscle Hypertrophy

We now know that humans, mice, and cattle can be born with a double dose of a genetic mutation in their muscle causing immense strength. The condition is called myostatin-related muscle hypertrophy. Both copies of a gene for a protein called myostatin are inactivated and the animals and humans grow up lean and so muscular that they are called "mighty, super, giant, etc." This explains why some people find it easy to get strong while others can lift weights day after day to little effect. The trait is genetic.

Since ancient times a Chinese master would carefully choose a student by screening his parents, grandparents, and their long lineage of ancestors to determine if the young student had any innate genetic potential. Then he would test them with extremely difficult poses, martial arts movement, and/or mental puzzles, in order to distinguish them, with certainty, from the average students. The "chosen" ones would be set aside for special training, becoming "private inner sanctum" students, and they became the next generation masters. The students lucky to have a genetic mutation were taught "secret skills and tricks" to reach their highest potential and became the super heroes we know today.

In the future you may be able to have your myostatin genes tested to decide whether to train to become a professional athlete.

Lever Power with Fast and Slow Twitch Muscle

What is it about elite sprinters that gives them the edge over non-sprinters? The length of an elite sprinter's heel is 25 percent shorter with toes one centimeter longer than non-sprinters, allowing them a functional lever to generate a more powerful push-off with a longer push against the running surface. Once the spring is sprung off the starting blocks, the sprinter continues with his blessing of fast-twitch muscle fibers.

You can usually determine through observation whether a child has a gene for greater fast or slow twitch muscles. You'll see explosive speed and power along with quick change-of-pace, stop-and-go movements. You can also have a genetic test for fast-twitch muscle which might imply your ability to excel in certain sports.

Paranormal Psychics with Special Energy Control

Paranormal psychic abilities are more difficult to recognize at a young age but, like physical traits, some people are born with extraordinary unique mental powers. Often the powers remain hidden until the person finds a friendly nurturing environment among other psychics who then help uncover the trait.

Epigenetics

Epigenetics is the branch of science that studies the way environmental factors alter the way our genes are expressed, making even identical twins different. It's now proven that our environment, including diet and lifestyle, can change the expression of our genes by influencing chemical switches within our cells collectively known as the epigenome. The first six years of life are most important to developing our personal belief system in how we function in the world, thus setting our baseline epigenome. Twins have been followed throughout their lives to prove gene expression is constantly shifting from baseline to fulfill the perceived needs of the individual. Some say we can create our future through the epigenome.

Science recently discovered that long-lived worms can transmit their extended lifespan to the next generation by passing on changes in the way their genes are used, rather than differences in DNA itself. A study has shown that nematode worms can inherit a "memory of longevity" from their parents even though their DNA remains unchanged. The worm has been a good model for humans and some believe the results of the study can be applied to ourselves.

"Epigenetic inheritance" is the process where organisms pass on changes in the way genes are used rather than in the genes themselves. It gives you the power to reprogram your cells. Some believe that's where the idea of using mental alchemy to bring your chi to a constant boil truly gives the effort its purpose. It's beautiful work and implies that epigenetic changes can carry across generations and we now realize that not everything is written in the genes. Plus, you can pass transgenerational epigenetic traits to your children as a result of persevering study with a guru. This inheritance can give your children a short-term advantage preparing them for the challenges that you are currently facing.

If you believe this then perfecting a martial arts move 100,000 times or standing in a balanced pose with intense mental heat for an hour, with the correct intention suited for your specific genetic make-up, may be a way to reprogram your cells to benefit you and your future lineage.

In summary, you can't change your dragon, but you can reprogram it to work more effectively during challenging times for both you and your progeny.

I hope this information encourages you to continue studying with your master but with a different, more practical, achievable, and satisfying goal. Life has more beauty and joy when you share your unique energetic strengths within your community. The sooner you discover your dragon and cultivate its innate talents, the greater your service to society. That's a goal worth having, plus achievable.

CHAPTER 19
YIN AIN'T YANG FITNESS

The Most Natural, Easy and Effective Way To Fitness, Health, Longevity and Moving Meditation…plus look and feel 5, 10, or even 20 years younger.

Imagine for a moment that you could plug into an exciting source of inner energy and flip on a switch that could reverse the aging process…even if you're already in your 60s, 70s, or 80s?

Imagine increased muscle and tendon strength, greater stamina, quicker reflexes and losing those extra pounds you've put on as the years have passed.

Imagine better balance, improved visual perception, a normal appetite with fewer food cravings, a more powerful immune system and the same peak metabolism you had before the cycle of aging crept in.

READ THIS NOW!

Because I've got a breakthrough answer for you that might be the

Anti-Aging Cure for the Common Birthday.

Dear Friend in Search of the Complete Life Path Package,

If you're like me and you suffered any kind of health challenge with mental and/or physical discomfort, I'm sure you've seen plenty of hype for programs that promise to rewire your body's hidden healing energy hardware. The marketplace is saturated with ridiculous overblown healing claims for exercise and meditation secrets.

These "miracle cures" are supposed to solve all the problems of a stress filled lifestyle by boosting your physical and mental reservoir of chi/energy—you know, that golden sweet honeydew nectar that flows within and without your being and is the creative force behind your existence.

Maybe you're one of the many, just like me, who have paid a small fortune for books, dvd's, seminars and personal instruction, hoping to finally find the answer to your inner quest for health and longevity. You rip open the package with eager anticipation... follow the instructions... and all you get is a few lost pounds, the slightest wriggle of struggling muscle fibers, and a trickle of a few warm swellings of chi.

Don't get me wrong. Everything on the market shelf for self-improvement has some benefit. But the simple fact is... nearly every program available today isn't addressing the whole system in a simple easy to do and understandable way.

Why? Because the scientific basis for health, fitness, and meditation is enormous. If you also include the esoteric teachings on the body, mind, and soul you would have an astoundingly complex infinite library of understandings.

Simply stated, most of the health and fitness programs today only work ONE THIRD of the puzzle. They focus on either the body, mind or spirit. Some combine TWO THIRDS by tying together body and mind. And the few that encompass ALL THREE—body, mind, and spirit—are so complex that few, if any, truly benefit and most students usually end up more confused and less healthy than when they started.

Many fitness enthusiasts spend 10, 20, 30 and even more years with regular workouts such as running, lifting, stretching, and punching. Others study more esoteric paths such as yoga, tai chi and meditation without even coming close to figuring it out.

Both types of seekers often end up with a shorter than normal life span suffering from physical breakdown and disease way before the young age of 55.

But I'm about to put an end to all that nonsense. I'm going to show you an ancient and forgotten but now considered "new" breakthrough exercise that can help you take care of all three treasures…in one convenient, gentle, and easy to understand exercise system that I call…Yin Ain't Yang Fitness.

With just one simple physical movement that I call "Vibrashake" and the slightest bit of mental focus using your teeth and jaws, you can immediately start the process of becoming intimately familiar with your body, mind and chi…and silence the nagging frustrations that other physical and mental systems of health and longevity burden you with.

Let me explain…

Many of you are already familiar with what I consider to be the "Best Body With Mind" exercise which is spotlighted on my website *www.Tooth-Fight.com*. This is a very serious Yang, hard driving, gut busting, mind blowing physical and mental workout…not for wimps!

Now I would like to give you the Yin aspect that will help you flip your inner switch to access the deep energy you need for any type of extreme muscle burning Yang exercise. You can call this the Best Body Without Mind exercise. It is more playful, childlike, enjoyable and better suited for the majority of today's busy and stressed out health and fitness enthusiasts. Yin Ain't Yang Fitness is the most effective exercise "without" mind because "no mind" is the best "no way" to relaxation, health, longevity and inner peace.

But if you're already a well conditioned weekend warrior don't think for a minute that a soft relaxed yin workout is any less important than a tough and rowdy yang workout because according to ancient teachings a healthy and fit long life is one where yin balances yang. Both are needed to maintain excellent health and fitness, one not being more important than the other.

So, for those looking for REAL punishment, I've developed the perfect complement to Vibrashake. I call it Die Chi For Dummies, a mind numbing, glute busting, tai chi based exercise using your mind, teeth jaws, and elementary tai chi principles.

Yin Ain't Yang Fitness featuring vibrashake is the simplest most effective exercise program for vigor, health, longevity and relaxed inner peace that can be enjoyed by any age group at any fitness level. Die Chi For Dummies is the next level up, for the fitness warrior thirsting for tai chi secrets and ready to martyr his beautiful body and mind for the quest toward unknowable ancient golden treasures.

Skyrocket your tai chi to i-CHI
INCREDIBLE — CENTERED — HARMONY — INFINITY

GET REAL WITH YOUR TAI CHI and FITNESS!
Take my "Tai-to-Die" 90 day challenge with a 100% money back guarantee and experience the remarkable benefits of "Yin Ain't Yang Fitness" for yourself!

CHAPTER 20
TAO TE TOOTH

Yoga unites the three treasures of Tai Chi—Beauty, Love, Spirit—however, joining the upper and lower teeth is the simplest path to understanding.

Bite, Chew, Eat... and Carry A Bright Belly.

The Tao of Grand Ultimate Teeth Is The Real Missing Link To Health.

Eat Like A Bird and Brush Your Beak. A Simple Way To Prevent A Toothless Tweet.

The Journey of a Thousand Steps in Extracting Energy and Nutrition from Food Begins with a Single Bite.

Your contentment in life reflects the degree of yin and yang in natural balance. Contentment is one measure by which we can gauge personal balance and growth. Is artificially whitening your teeth for fame and fortune a dysfunctional impulse or a useful exercise increasing contentment? A wise person carefully reflects on his methods for achieving long term goals.

Let the workings of your smile remain a mystery, just show people the result.

A Master need ask only one simple question to lead a student to knowing... "what do you know?" The correct response will reflect an opening and flowing of all the Qi meridians of the body into a more natural way.

A missing tooth is a blessing that leads you to search for oneness with the universe, hoping to build a bridge between two teeth and the heavens in between.

Those who know don't talk, but watch out for their bite.

Tai chi reveals the dust of stumbling confusion remaining on the surface of your mind's mirror. Toothbrushing is an on-going effort to unscramble the confusion of microbial dental plaque from the surface of your tooth.

A warm smile can melt the coldest heart.

Digest large tissues and minerals by first reducing them into small liquid particles. Deal with difficult foods by using temperature and pressure to break them down into easily absorbed nourishment.

Any food that enters the masticatory universe of your mouth returns to the common fertile source in the earth.

It is fitting for a great denture to suction up.

Cultivate tooth Qi with caution; at the beginning imagine your tooth has the strength of a strong egg shell. Keep the tongue out of harm's way, as if surrounded by poison tipped spears.

The mouth becomes exhausted if you chew too fast and bite too often with great force. Better to first slowly and thoroughly moisten your food with enzymatic saliva.

Hard teeth and soft tongue complement each other. The more your tongue moves the food bolus, the more your teeth produce digestible nutrition.

Ordinary people think very little about their teeth. Some actually find them useless and prefer to replace them with artificial dentures.

If teeth were the kind of thing ordinary people thought was useful besides just for eating, for example, as a means to become one with the Tao, dentists would have disappeared long ago.

Today a wise man barely knows his wisdom teeth, and if that sounds paradoxical try making sense of the Tao Te Ching.

One must not blame a blemish on your tooth for your discontent. Many cosmetic dental enhancements are merely obstructions that hinder your progress.

A smile lights up your tan-tiens.

Meditative tai chi is a road map for getting lost in the Tao; reading signs is useful but directions not needed.

Teeth and gums are genetically cut into your DNA. It is the emptiness between the upper and lower oral segments that make the teeth and gums useful.

Healthy teeth last a lifetime if the intention behind their purpose is survival of the organism.

If you're lost in Tao and don't remember which direction is up, try smiling and follow the corners of your mouth.

The softer tongue is like the general of an army. Once the food is engaged behind the lips and surrounded with teeth, the tongue strategizes the battle and cajoles the enemy/food into tooth traps for slicing, tearing, and grinding.

We desire to understand the functioning of our mouth through research and experimentation, hoping to uncover the unseen, but these revelations are only the surface effects of deep subtle energy.

The value of a tooth lies in its location, the value of a tongue lies in its reliability, the value of their interdependence lies in a generous spirit.

Never underestimate the biting task at hand. If you do you could cripple both tooth and tongue.

The oral cavity is an esoteric system built on a holistic view of reality. It unifies all existence within and around us. The upper and lower teeth represent the duality of all phenomena as an opposing manifestation of the same fundamental function of mastication.

Taoism regards Nature as the model of true reality. In the natural world all effort is devoted to survival. In humans the most basic instinct for survival is in the teeth, tongue, and jaws.

The Tao is not about becoming perfect. A Sage practicing Taoism has never been so wise and perfect to have never bit his own tongue.

Each tooth in your mouth has an individual purpose working toward a unified goal of the organism. Alone, each tooth is ineffective. All 32 teeth voluntarily submit to social behavior which benefits the organism without sacrificing the original potential of the individual tooth.

Lao Tzu's philosophy of "non-interference" is inherently demonstrated in the flawless eruption of the teeth into perfect occlusion. It is not wise to waste precious time attempting to improve minor variations in tooth intercuspation that may not bring tangible personal benefits. Usually, dental harmony will be achieved by allowing the natural rhythms of the oral cavity unlimited freedom of expression during guided visualization.

Our baby milk teeth are grown into our mouth for a short time to better prepare ourselves to mortal reality. The theory of tao infers that permanent teeth are the surviving entity which if healthy, like the soul, means that a better life on earth provides a better afterlife. The duality of physical and spiritual are complimentary and totally bound.

Mastication, the biting chewing and eating of food, reminds one that life is a struggle, a fundamental underlying assumption in Taoism's prescription for a healthy and long life.

A toothbrush, dental floss, interdental pick/brush, and tongue scraper are tools of specific Taoist principles important for maintaining the physical body, the house of the soul.

Life is a constant exchange of yin and yang. The dentist gives you gold tooth fillings while taking gold coins from your checkbook. He extracts a painful abscessed tooth and you gain a pain-free night's sleep.

An inward smile is the shortest distance between you and the Tao.

Every individual tooth possesses its own vibrational frequency which is associated with the inherent Qi energy determined by the alignment at the time of eruption. Orthodontic alignment serves as a channel of cosmic energy within each person. The flow of energy affects one's fate and in the case of crooked, missing, displaced, and extra teeth, it should be the objective of the orthodontist to realign an individual's personal teeth Qi with that of the Cosmos to correct any misalignment caused by embryonic confusion from metaphysical forces.

*In understanding the link between the mind and body, you must rec-
ognize the mind controls the body. The two are interdependent,
but mental control is of the utmost importance. Your mind should
not let your teeth chatter away mindlessly. A confused mind issues incorrect commands that may cause the human dentition to
grind itself senseless while traveling through life's stressful cycles.
This is diagnosed as bruxism. When the mind is overworked it
becomes worried, and worry contributes to bruxism. A spiritual
person can navigate through life's dangerous waters by allowing
a clear mind to make correct decisions, therefore eliminating the
possibility for harmful tooth clenching and grinding.*

*Taoism encourages "stillness" as a way to clear the muddy waters
of runaway thoughts that block a crystal clear view of reality.
Meditation is a process that helps you rid yourself of confused
thoughts with dysfunctional value. It is the mental equivalent of
tooth brushing and flossing away harmful dental plaque colonies.
When your external senses and oral microbiology are disturbed,
you should rest your mind and seek tranquility inside. Brushing
and flossing is a practical solution by which you can turn on your
senses and shut down your brain, to some degree, for a rest. In
essence, you teach your brain how to not think yet still be awake
while performing oral hygiene, a skill which can be transferred to
other activities during your wakeful day.*

*Meditation is focused visualization and it is most definitely work, but
in a relaxed way, especially beneficial during oral hygiene practices. Focusing on work with specific intention, such as brushing
teeth and visualizing the teeth becoming brighter, prevents the
mind from wandering to some other competing thoughts.*

Western dental medicine is now beginning to recognize that most dental disease can be traced to physical, microbiological, and biochemical imbalances triggered by mental dysfunction. Treating the worldly imbalances can temporarily alleviate the symptoms of disease, but reduction of mental stress while balancing the energetic Qi meridians yields far greater long lasting physical benefits.

The dental chair is a microcosm of the universe where false teeth dentures are made from the the void of toothlessness.

An attacking mouth with a biting force of 1000 pounds can be deflected with only a one ounce poke of a numbing needle.

A true smile is a spiritual connection to original source.

A healthy diet of Tao is found somewhere within a peaceful state of mind, usually right before or after a daily exercise of finding and following your mission in life, always exchanging at least three pounds of fatty frowns with three pounds of lean smiles.

Visit your dentist because he can guide you toward that one bite into the perfect occlusion of Tao.

The law of action/reaction states that every drilling zing to tooth has a corresponding screaming z-yikes!

The Tao of Tooth is mother to both the harmony of structured alignment and chaos in bruxism.

If your teeth cleaning is a stressful occurrence it's because your feeble mind isn't relaxed enough to understand the complex inside out situation of your dental hygienist, deep in meditation, being disturbed with a splash in her face by your self-assertive sublingual salivary glands from under your uncompromising cantankerous fluttering tongue.

To avoid fits of depression a dentist must gaze beyond the characteristic change and decay of his patient's secret oral universe.

It is profitless to launch a mission of mercy while a civil war is boiling in the oral cavity, as a tooth in conflict and in the heat of infection cannot be conveniently approached from any direction. Decay, blood and pus protect it from courageous dentists furnished with unsuitable equipment which can inflict more harm than good. First organize a small furtive force of drugs and herbs to creep into the main arteries and wait for their report.

In darkness, clear vision begins with a single point of light that illuminates your being with clash and flash. Spark the light of your inner smile...teeth not required...and the way reveals itself.

END BOOK
YIN AIN'T YANG
The Ancient Way to Better Health

Bite Deep Into The Mystery of Yin Ain't Yang

Looking for some jaw-dropping tooth-breaking news that could take you higher than laughing gas? Bite into this book in the right place, with the right intention, and in harmony with your imagination, and you could unlock jaw-locking secrets. That's why I didn't release this book in an e-book format. Biting into an e-reader would set you up for a possible jaw-breaking tooth shattering experience. That would be worse than dental drilling without a shot of tooth-numbing juice.

So, unmuzzle your bite and stop getting your teeth kicked in. Bite deep into the mystery of Yin Ain't Yang, literally, in the right way, for a Richter Scale 9.0 toothquake revelation. Email me for more details at *info@revolutiontooth.com*.

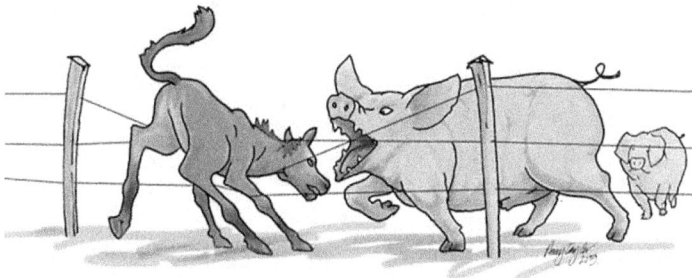

Teeth in Mortal Combat

How To Unleash Your Basic Instinct For Survival

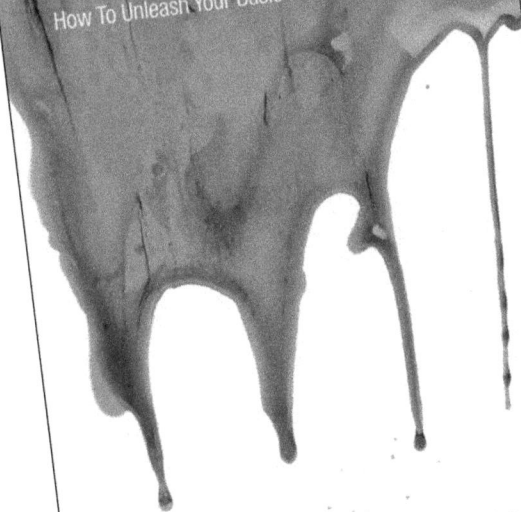

Lester Sawicki, DDS

TEETH
IN MORTAL
COMBAT

HOW TO Unleash Your Basic Instinct FOR SURVIVAL

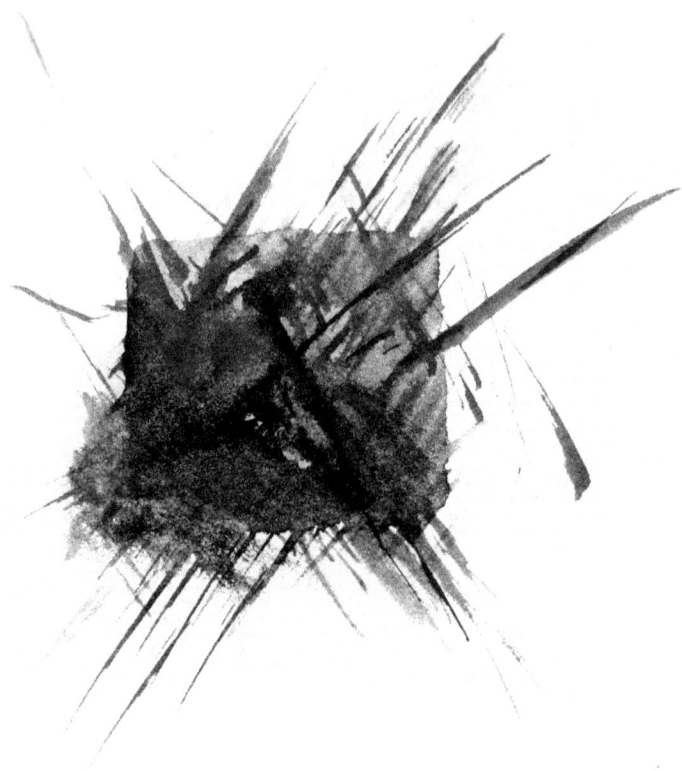

PREFACE

As a seasoned practitioner of martial arts and meditation—and a student of the connection between healthy teeth and a vibrant long life—I asked myself what bearing teeth had on my martial arts and meditation practice. A series of small, serendipitous thoughts led to personal insights which further ignited a powerful epiphany. In many respects, this epiphany was as shocking as it was enlightening, and the thought processes involved were somewhat radical and 'outside of the box.'

Mark my words in this: the conformist shackles his self-progress. The open-minded rebel cuts a path of discovery with a sword honed by hard questions. Therefore, I dare not add to the dust on your mirror. The few words I use will not place you in harm's way, and the following dissertation will be brief, painted within a fog of misty clouds. The fiery sun within you is more than capable of burning through these humble, perhaps meaningless revelations. The only advice given is that you FIGHT tooth and nail to Lift the Veil of Mystery.

Lifting the Veil of Mystery is a ritual practiced by all would be martial artists. You have chosen this moment in time to be here with me, to catch a glimpse behind the veil. I honor you for that, and will share some of my very personal experiences and treasures discovered in the practice of martial arts: Perfection as a goal can paralyze movement. The path is a journey of error. Questions chisel away the multiple coverings of fear; by becoming aware of one's fear, transformation can happen; fear does not transform into its opposite, bravery; when you accept your fear, the transformation is respect for your power and the fear slowly disappears. To become a Master—"There is no answer."

In my opinion, the blinding snow laden mountains of martial art styles, as some may claim, do not have a unifying original source. There is no single rooted tree of self-defense from which all the others sprang and branched out. We find no one movement that is simple, pure, undiluted, and therefore, more powerful and effective than all the others. What we do find in the turbulent, snowy, wind-swept mountain peaks is Stillness—from which all forms arise. It has no name.

Think of a wintry blue sky thick with snow clouds that condense and crystallize the first original snowflakes. Which snowflake hits the solid earth first to hold the distinction of being the Authentic One? Is that the 'snowflake' we should try to emulate in our martial arts fighting style? Is that the singular form that holds the superior wisdom, strength, and effectiveness we are searching for? Clouds do not vie for the title of "Creator of First Snowflake," nor do snow flakes fall from the sky competing to be the first to land on earth. It is IMPOSSIBLE to imagine the very first snowflake that gently touched earth's highest mountain peak. Were humans there to discover, preserve, and catalog it? Who today can claim and prove direct lineage to this venerable form? Yet importantly, the snow crystals do, in their floating dance downward to solid ground, travel together. They all grow in synchrony, each having a unique and intricate design with recognizable symmetry.

And likewise with martial arts, I believe we waste precious time arguing one fighting style's superiority over another. There is no single original martial art that is more effective and deadly than those that have followed. There is no one movement that defeats all others. When discussing and comparing various martial art styles, you might as well be talking about snowflakes.

What piques my curiosity is that something appears to exist behind the common symmetry of all martial arts styles. For lack of a better word, I call it "instinct." Humans today still depend on instinct for survival; it is the basis for all self-defense when engaged in Mortal Combat. And in this book I reveal an instinct common to all, from infant to adult. It is this distinct instinct that sparks all the necessary forces needed to recreate human life. Beginning at birth it feeds, protects, and preserves us until the day we decide to pass from this earth ... This instinct, along with many more pearls of information, is revealed in this book where you will discover Survival Instincts Hidden Behind the Secret Smile of Laughing Buddha. As an added hidden bonus, you will learn why I believe "Molar Combat with Killer White Teeth and Massive Jaws" may be a Secret to Immortality.

Based on my own experience, I believe society can depress, deform, corrupt, and mutate an individual's elemental expression of instinct. Instinct breathes life into the symmetry that exists in all of us, yet today dwells suppressed, crippled, or dormant in most of us. In this book I try to illuminate and release our birthright to an instinct nearly buried today among society's artificial constructs. I hope that after reading this book you will have a greater understanding of what it means to truly live FREE as a human being—with the freedom to express your most basic instinct for survival.

I sincerely hope that the turbulent joys and sorrows that have arisen from my twenty-five year study of the mysteries of the East will benefit you many times over.

Lester Sawicki, DDS

PROLOGUE

If you are one of the hundreds of thousands of aspiring martial artists studying hard under the tutelage of a Master, you have most certainly heard and read the following tenets many times:

A.) The lowest level of victory over an opponent is through the use of muscular strength alone.

B.) The middle level utilizes and releases one's intrinsic energy, or chi, as a kite on a string.

C.) At the highest level one projects the spirit at the opponent and they therefore dare not take any aggressive action.

Some Martial Art Masters in the United States of America have a rule of thumb stating that it takes twenty years of consistent practice in each of the three levels in order to boil the cauldron of ignorance into the steam of wizardry. That means a minimum of sixty years of consistent, methodical, focused, blood, guts, sweat, and tears training is required in the pursuit of Lifting the Veil of Mystery.

In my experience and observation over the last fifty years, few Americans (myself included) have gone beyond a mere warming of the pot in level "A." Many have become sick, disabled, or died during their quest for Mastery of level "B" (sadly, some were friends). I am sure that you will also agree that Level "C" has been reduced for the majority to nothing more than myths exchanged over beer, coffee, and healing teas.

But it is worth noting that some of the Asian Masters who travel to the West to demonstrate and teach martial arts are not bound by this Twenty Year Golden Rule of Time. Many of them—some under the age of thirty-five and a few barely in their late teens—can readily demonstrate all three levels. What is the truth behind mastering the three levels? Where are the answers?

Many mysteries may be solved in states of deep relaxation and heavy dreams. I should not have been surprised then, when it was during such a state that my cauldron began to lightly steam, misting a few fleeting answers to my conscious mind. The veil of mystery began to flutter, if not lift. But I was surprised—AND angry! The scenario was not presenting itself as expected. In fact, the whole scene seemed to be running in reverse. However, my experience gleaned from scars scalded by burning sweat—in concert with these revelations—helped to transmute my anger into the discovery of Hex-Diamond White Teeth & Predator X Jaw and the realization that they are critical to mastering a long life and perhaps even another path to immortality.

I cannot claim that the reading of this book will make your path toward enlightenment any easier or quicker. My prayer is that it brings into your life blossoms of a more fragrant flower!

PART ONE

GATHERING STORM CLOUDS

CHAPTER 1
ORIGINAL CHI

Evolutionists contend that man is descended from prehistoric creatures of sea, sky, and land. The first martial artists were profound philosophers who understood this long ago. The innate energy of each animal was visualized and meditated upon by the first Masters. They devised the Animal Form fighting styles in order to imitate and learn from these creatures, as each animal has specialized instincts for survival that are perfect for that animal's body shape, build, capability, and personality. They learned that studying and practicing Animal Forms could activate latent but powerful animal instincts embedded in man's DNA.

After much dedicated study and practice, an animal's natural power may be tapped to invigorate the practitioner's chi. What was once dormant, due to societal constraints, becomes a vital force behind the martial artist's expression of chi. If one can engage all of the animal energy within oneself, a formidable warrior emerges. One must dive deep into the bubbling well of animal forms to locate the source, but if one pays homage to it, the being quickens and everything seems possible. All dangers dissolve.

Let us review some of the animal forms.

> Dragon
> Tiger
> Snake
> Crane
> Leopard
> Deer

Monkey
Bear
Elephant
Lion
Horse

All of these animals, with the exception of the crane, use their teeth and jaws in combat. And the crane, of course, uses its beak to stab. Elephants use teeth and tusks. The tusks are actually specialized upper incisors, or front teeth, and the elephant has six teeth which are replaced several times throughout its life, a characteristic shared with sharks. Deer have surprisingly powerful bites and, having latched on to their opponent, shake their heads and tear in the manner of pit bulls. The Komodo Dragon, the world's largest lizard, delivers a powerful bite with its serrated teeth and it has been recently discovered that they also utilize a powerful venom to bring down their victims. Monkeys maul with their canines and front teeth. Horses are also tenacious biters.

And it is an undeniable fact that in the early ages of mankind, formidable teeth and jaws were often crucial for survival. Teeth functioned as tools to help create body coverings as animal hides were softened by working the teeth and jaws. Self-defense often depended on the most basic weapon—sharp teeth and strong jaws—long before man learned to build weapons. Yet to this day, men, women and children will use their teeth and jaws in mortal combat to best their assailant, be it man or beast.

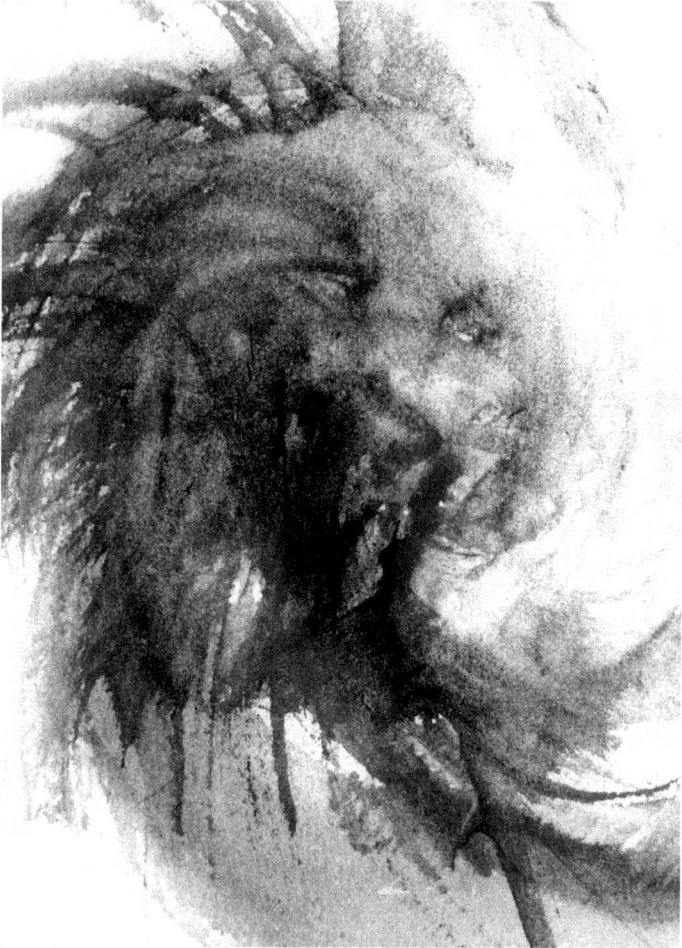

CHAPTER 2
TEETH — OUR MOST PRIMITIVE AND PRIMARY WEAPONS OF CHOICE?

1. Teeth are Man's Most Basic Weapon

In the human race, teeth have always been an important component of our weaponry. The information presented here explains man's basic instinct for survival through the use of our oldest and most natural means of self-defense—our teeth and jaws.

Mortal Combat is the term applied to violence associated with life and death struggles. During Mortal Combat, there are moments when the teeth are often the ONLY available and effective weapon that can provide distraction, inflict injury, and even cause death. Teeth can inflict mortal injury when applied to the exposed vital anatomy of the trachea (windpipe) and jugular vein. Teeth are also used to inflict serious injury during sexual attacks such as rape or child abuse, sometimes leading to homicide. In these cases, the assailant uses the bite as an expression of dominance, rage, and bestial insanity. And all too often teeth may be the last, or— only, line of defense in case of attack. Wise is the dentist who recognizes your teeth as such effective weaponry and he might do well to offer you dental treatment options that enhance your teeth for times of Mortal Combat.

Today, one would be hard pressed to find a martial arts school that covers the usage of teeth in Mortal Combat. One might question the necessity of teaching something that is basically a hardwired instinctive reflex. The answer is that the average person has had his/her energy pathway to the teeth and jaw blocked in some way and to some degree. This handicap inhibits the resourceful utilization of the *"dental fright/flight response"* involving the use of teeth and jaw. The possible causes of this energetic disturbance will be covered shortly. But first, a discussion about a side effect of energy restriction in the human bite instinct—Bruxism.

2. Bruxism and Teeth Sharpening

Bruxism is an involuntary, non-functional, rhythmic gnashing, grinding, and clenching of teeth—not including chewing movements—of the mandible. It is a subconscious, parafunctional condition that occurs either during stage 2 sleep or while awake. It may be secondary to anxiety, tension, or dental problems due to stress or drugs.

Bruxism activity occurs in most humans at some time in their lives. The prevalence of clenching is reported to be twenty percent, whereas sleep grinding is seen in six percent of the adult general population. It often leads to loss of tooth enamel surface, cracking of teeth, headaches, mouth and facial pain, jaw pain, and limited jaw movement.

The cause of bruxism is not completely agreed upon. Today, the general consensus among dentists is that bruxism is a pathological process intrinsically related to the dentition and/or musculature of the head and neck. If the teeth are not positioned correctly (malocclusion), the pointed anatomical cusps interfere with normal jaw movement. During function, the muscles of mastication overwork to compensate for the interferences. The muscular tension that results will eventually cause or contribute to:

- Earache
- Insomnia
- Headache
- Tooth pain

- Depression
- TMJ joint pain
- Eating disorders
- Sore or painful jaw
- Head and neck muscle pain
- Anxiety, stress, and tension

Daily stress may also trigger bruxism dependent on the level of stress, diet, sleep habits, posture, and the ability to relax. Once again, stress related muscle activation and over-use is intrinsically causal for the jaws to clench and grind the teeth

The relation of bruxism to the theory of thegosis is quite interesting. *Thegosis (meaning to whet or sharpen) describes the sharpening of anterior teeth under specific conditions, some of which may be related to social situations.* Dr. Ronald Every introduced thegosis in the 1960's to prove that bruxism is a sociological pathology. This means that a psycho-emotional driven solution rather than a physical dental/muscular cure must be examined. He presented good evidence that primitive man's behavioral trait of clenching to strengthen jaw muscles, and grinding to sharpen teeth for self-defense, may be the basis of clinical teeth grinding.

Most dentists today treat bruxism from a physical dental/ muscular direction and prescribe palliative measures to help relax the spastic muscles involved. The treatment involves a physical device such as a night guard or bite splint. This may be accompanied by massage, chiropractic manipulation, biofeedback, hot-cold therapy, far infrared light, acupuncture, acupressure, hypnosis, nutrition, herbs, etc.

Very few dental professionals accept or treat bruxism as a psychosocial pathology. Dr. Every was not able to win many supporters for his theory of thegosis, even though he spent over thirty years analyzing and presenting convincing historical data to the scientific world. I believe part of the obstacle to the acceptance of his ideas is the fact that dentists choose their profession because they like to work with their hands. They love drilling, bridging, implanting, broaching, rotor-rooting, root canaling, grafting, carving, shaping, brushing, painting, etching, bonding, slathering, smoothing, polishing, and glossing teeth. Ask a dentist to sit down and talk about emotional psychosocial pathology in relation to bruxism, and be prepared for blank stares as he hides his furious and desperately twisting fingers from your vision, constructing a midair dream of his next patient's fixed cosmetic enhancement.

Thegosis would likely be more accepted if dentists could be convinced of the benefits in connecting with their own life force/chi, and then, through that lens, using their chi to examine the source of bruxism. Once one establishes one's own reconnection of chi to the teeth and jaws, connecting the dots from bruxism to muscle building and teeth sharpening is mere child's play.

Paleontologists may never find enough convincing evidence of teeth sharpening in humans, but the chi never lies about the past. We need only interpret the results of our own investigation with wisdom and maturity.

This is my challenge to all dentists: *Let us connect with our chi, come to know and understand it, and use it to help our patients overcome their patterns of disease and pathology simultaneously on all levels—physical, mental, and spiritual.*

3. The Growth and Development of Teeth for Slicing Large Chunks

Dr. Every defined thegosis as *"sharpening a tooth, beak or bill by deliberately and forcefully grinding it across surfaces of an opposing tooth, beak or bill."* It is used by many vertebrate and invertebrate animals in order to sharpen the teeth for use as tools and/or weapons. Some examples are:

- Rat
- Sheep
- Baboon
- Sea urchin
- Vampire bat
- Hippopotamus

Dr. Every theorized that humans grind their teeth with the evolutionary purpose of honing the incisors to a sharp edge for cutting and slicing in battle. Thegosis also strengthens the primary muscles used for biting in self-defense—the masseter and temporalis. It takes only a couple days of clenching to rapidly pump up the biting muscle fibers, enabling a stronger, deeper, and more lethal bite. This process is called the *"dental aspect of the fright/flight response"* and may have enhanced the survival odds of early humans.

In order to better understand teeth sharpening within the theory of thegosis, we should follow the growth and development of human teeth beginning with birth.

An infant is born toothless in order to more efficiently suckle at the mother's breast. As the child matures, the teeth erupt to help break down solid food and this initiates the child's eventual separation from the mother. The child must then strengthen its muscles of mastication to begin self-feeding at nature's table.

When an infant is born, the entire gut, including the colon, is sterile. However, as the baby's head begins to slide through the vagina, bacteria are picked up on the infant's lips. When it suckles on the mother's nipple, more bacteria are swallowed with the milk. As the baby begins to eat more solid food, pre-chewing transfers even more bacteria to the intestinal flora. The mother must pass to the child her own prebiotic and probiotic bacteria necessary to digest solid food and enhance immunity to disease. This is a normal and desirable sequence of events.

Nature originally intended the mother to chew, soften, and transfer predigested food to the child's mouth. This teaches the child with newly erupting teeth to safely chew and swallow solid food without aspirating whole particles and choking to death. Pre-chewing food is no longer a part of today's modern culture, but it is a practice still seen in poor, developing countries. Why take the time to chew your baby's food when you can buy a jar of commercially blended baby food at the local grocery store? I'm joking, of course!

Mother's milk is BY FAR the most potent source of nutrition, minerals, and vitamins for the infant. It is also the very best source of prebiotics and probiotics for the brand new bacteria factory in the baby's colon. Infant formula manufacturers have been forever trying to replicate mother's milk, but nothing comes close to what a mother's natural milk and saliva does to create a healthy environment in the baby's colon. Likewise, commercially blended baby food could NEVER replace the healthy benefits of pre-chewing.

Science has shown that the infant's health is directly affected by that of the mother, beginning with its life as an embryo. Infants who are breastfed and whose mothers consumed foods containing prebiotics or took prebiotic supplements, both before and after birth, have much fewer and less intense allergies as they mature. A natural childbirth through the vagina, in addition to breastfeeding, provides the infant with healthier gut bacterial colonization than those who are born by cesarean and are fed commercial formulas.

However, it is best to use caution if you consider pre-chewing your baby's food, as beneficial as well as harmful bacteria are transferred from mother to child. Mothers should make every effort to stay healthy in all physical and mental respects. The infant's health is affected, for better and worse, by bacteria and viruses that are passed between mother and child. Healthy vaginal and oral inoculation of the infant remains a prominent marker of good health, even into adulthood and beyond. Passing harmful bacteria and viruses can promote disease and life-threatening medical issues even in the adult years. There has been one verified case of a mother passing the AIDS virus to her child by pre-chewing food. Mothers pass along as many as five hundred different species of bacteria and viruses, including those that cause tooth decay, gum disease, hepatitis B, hepatitis C and Group B streptococcus, among others. If a woman is planning on having children, she should be aware of this and do everything possible to improve her own health before becoming pregnant. Newborn babies deserve every chance for a normal, healthy, disease-free life.

As previously discussed, one of the reasons humans have teeth is to facilitate complete separation from the mother. This is part of a logical progression and schedule, all related to the eruption of the baby's teeth. Let's now examine the role teeth play in the theory of thegosis.

Deciduous (baby) teeth are smaller, with thinner protective enamel, and have less prominent cusp tips compared to adult teeth. Their main purpose is help the child make the transition from liquid breast milk to softer food solids. Logically, the smaller mouth and less developed muscles of the growing child influence the appropriate size and shape of tooth to perfectly chew the next stage of soft food solids. Baby teeth are "pint-sized" compared to full-sized adult teeth. The baby is not yet strong enough or experienced in safe technique to tackle hard, tough foods it would find in its environment. It has to remain attached to the mother a little longer. Evolution has mandated tiny baby teeth for the child as the best size and strength for the job at hand.

At about twelve years of age, the child's deciduous teeth have been replaced by twenty-eight fully formed adult sized teeth. The child has become a young adult with a larger, muscled body, and stronger, thicker, enameled teeth. Psychologically and physically the young adult is ready to freely begin feasting at nature's table. At this stage of development, the teenager is also ready to prepare for the more advanced and formidable adult task of using his/her teeth as tools and weapons.

Many children today are reaching physical and sexual maturity earlier than in the past, although emotional maturity does not seem to be following this trend. American girls in the year 1800 had their first period, on average, at about age 17. By 1900 that had dropped to 14. Now it is 12. *Some scientists attribute early physical maturation to spilled and dumped chemical hormones polluting our water and food systems. I myself have seen pre-teens with their full complement of thirty-two adult teeth, including wisdom teeth. This phenomena has come about within the past twenty-five years, whereas previously the average age for wisdom tooth eruption was between seventeen and twenty-two years of age.*

At this point, teeth sharpening needs to begin in order to help the young adult survive a long healthy life. Although the adult teeth are larger than deciduous, they still have relatively rounded incisor edges and cusp tips. The teeth, at this stage of development, need to be sharpened, and the jaw muscles bulked up, for efficient use as a tool for holding, cutting, molding, and softening clothing materials. They also need to be strengthened and sharpened for self-defense, in the Spirit of the Warrior.

More scientific information on the architecture of the tooth and how it becomes stronger with grinding, clenching, and tapping will be found in later chapters. But at this time, it is important to insist that readers of this text **must not attempt to sharpen and strengthen teeth without correct instruction and guidance.** *In other words: Don't do this at home.*

When chewing we grind, squeeze, break, cut, slice, chop, split, crack, crush, flake, stab, gash, and nick the food. Very few children today display advanced proficiency in all of these functions. I have never heard of a child under the age of twelve who can use their teeth to crack whole walnuts and chew through large bones. It takes an adult with adult teeth to demonstrate these minor achievements. When primitive man pushed his teeth beyond what was necessary for normal everyday function, as a tool and as a weapon in Mortal Combat, it required a strength and cutting edge MANY times more powerful and sharp than a child could manage. Children with baby teeth would be unable meet such advanced challenges.

I believe in the premise of thegosis, where primitive adults probably made a conscious effort to sharpen and strengthen the teeth and jaws, whereas today we brux subconsciously. In primitive society, the conscious sharpening and clenching action would have enabled the teeth to be a more effective tool for fashioning garments and processing food during mastication. Clenching would also prepare men and women for self-defense by strengthening the muscles involved in grasping, attacking, and protecting. The process would have sharpened the incisor front teeth to allow a lethal bite.

Humans have a more complex anatomy and arrangement of teeth. We use our front incisor teeth mainly for slicing/scissoring and the posterior molars for grinding. The incisors and canine capture and/or segment the prey/food. The anatomy of the premolars and molars shows cusps that serve to puncture food; crests that connect cusps to shear; and basins which crush or grind food. Humans also have shorter canines than other primates. We can easily sharpen our incisors and make side-slicing actions (like using scissors) with our front teeth because our canines do not interfere. This slicing action allows us to take large chunks out of food, prey, and assailants during self-defense. All other primates use their canines as a piercing weapon instead because their canines' longer length restricts the ability to slice sideways and segment the food.

Most carnivores use their enlarged and blade-like carnassial (fourth upper premolar and first lower molar) teeth for shearing flesh and bone in a scissoring, slicing, chopping, or shearing manner. When a dog or cat brings the side of its head up against a bone on which it is gnawing, it is probably using its carnassials.

4. Teeth as Weapons

Combatants today seldom use their teeth in fighting, especially to separate and remove a large chunk of flesh in one action. This is called a "segmentative bite" and is unique to humans, not seen in primates. This aspect of our jaws and dentition is what gives us a powerful advantage over other animals during combat. Our incisor bite force is remarkably powerful—comparable to that of many predators—and our ability to slice sideways can cause vicious lacerations. Many of us have seen the power of human teeth and jaws as aptly demonstrated by martial artists pulling multi-ton vehicles with their teeth, and many are undoubtedly familiar with the story of the Chinese burglar who could bite through iron bars.

Examining bruxism through the lens of thegosis makes good sense to me, and I believe further research into thegotic theory is warranted. In today's world, teeth grinding and clenching during subconscious bruxism may be interpreted as the chronic result of social conditioning to suppress, or repress, instinctive aggression. Many people today are failing to deal with psychosocial and emotional stressors that perpetuate defensive behaviors. This purportedly explains why stress is such a common factor in people who experience elevated levels of bruxism, particularly at night when they are asleep and not suppressing those emotions. People feel under attack, so subconsciously sharpen their teeth to defend themselves. One can make a strong a priori case for human teeth being used as weapons by our earliest ancestors. Today, however, for a variety of reasons, the growth and development of our teeth and jaws for use as a weapon has been stunted.

One reason for this is man's invention of, and modern dependence on, sophisticated weaponry. The relatively non-lethal hand has become more important with the introduction of artificial weapons such as club, knife, bow, gun, etc. Emphasis on survival has been deflected from the simple instinctual use of mouth, teeth, and jaws to the more superior, complex manipulation and coordination of hand-held weapons. The "open hand" needs formal training to develop into a deadly weapon. Warriors are trained in the deadly use of hand combat to police and protect the social congregation. This kind of organizational control helps maintain the species. Today, more than ever, "closed hand" cutting-edge military weapons require advanced training in use.

Societal restrictions on the use of the hands by warriors is almost non-existent, save for eye gouging, but society does place restrictions on the use of teeth. This is because, in the untrained human, the teeth are more lethal than the hand. The use of biting to kill does not need to be taught, as everyone possesses this instinct for survival. Biting is extremely dangerous and many of our ancestors undoubtedly perished as the result of infection due to virulent oral bacterial flora acquired through biting during combat. Taboos were placed on aggressive actions with teeth in order to preserve the population and growth of the community and in order to prevent chaos, death, and depopulation. Taboos on fighting with the teeth were also put in place by ancient dictators for reasons that will be examined in later chapters.

5. Modern Man's Teeth are Weak Compared to Those of Primitive Man

We no longer have warriors who use their teeth as weapons. Our crooked teeth and relatively weak jaws are almost never used in a life and death struggle. We rarely read about a person biting in self-defense as one last desperate attempt for survival. These facts usually remain hidden in autopsy reports and the media has little stomach for printing such shocking stories. But *why* has man almost entirely ceased to use teeth as weapons?

Paleontologists have studied primitive skulls and, for the most part, all artifacts show sufficient room for the normal thirty-two tooth dentition. Bite malocclusion appears to have been rare in ancient man, whereas today bite malocclusion is common. Studies have shown that the mean bite force of children changes with the occlusion (position of the teeth in the arch). Malocclusion (crooked teeth) results in weakened bite force. This is likely another possible reason why humans today rely less on their teeth during self-defense. Some researchers investigating the record high incidences of malocclusion in children believe that genetics and environmental factors play an important role.

We know that nutrition in the foetal stage affects the determination of tooth size. Increased tooth size is related to increased consumption of protein and fat in the modern diet. Vitamin and mineral deficient diets, along with hormone disruptors found in food and water supplies, lead to smaller bone growth, including the jaw. Larger teeth and smaller, more constricted jawbones leave less space for the teeth to erupt into their correct position and results in crooked teeth and weaker biting power.

The growth of the chewing apparatus may be affected by the eating behavior of children from infancy through puberty. It is known that bottle fed babies have a weaker structure and function of the jaw biting apparatus compared to babies who are breast fed. People who eat coarsely milled staple grains have more developed jaw muscle structure than those who eat a softer diet. Another factor that affected bite force in primitive man was the clenching of teeth and chewing on twigs, leaves, gum, and meat jerky—processes that can develop the masseter muscle, the driving force for biting. People who clench and chew on hard substances develop more muscle fibers in the masseter, resulting in greater jaw strength. Because of our processed fast-food diet, we chew less and the things we chew are softer. People also do not have, or are unable to make, the time to eat at a leisurely pace and chew their food thoroughly. And the result is that modern man's biting apparatus is weak in comparison with the diamond-steel teeth and massive jaws of our ancient relatives.

Another modern phenomena that contributes to weaker dentition is the preponderance of wisdom tooth extractions. As our brains continue to evolve and enlarge, our jawbones are becoming reduced in size to make more room within the skull. Genetic and environmental factors also explain why less dependence on the teeth and jaws for daily living leads to smaller jaw bones in humans and constricted room for wisdom teeth.

I hope that I have put forth enough theory, ideas, and opinions to illustrate my premise that our teeth, *rather than our hands,* remain our most primitive and primary weapons of choice. It is almost unheard of these days for a human to aggressively or defensively bite a fatally vulnerable neck. We repress our instincts and no longer have the sharp teeth and commanding jaws that would confidently bring us victory in battle. Instead, the modern one-on-one battle between warriors usually comprises high tech hand weapons such as guns or knives.

Later chapters in this book will continue to reveal how our society artificially controls and restricts the use of teeth in their ultimate, basic, instinctive use for self-defense. Historical evidence for this tragedy is not likely to surface, and the true reasons will probably remain buried and unknown, but the effects on humankind are obvious. Solutions to correct this current deficiency in the fight for survival during mortal combat are forthcoming.

CHAPTER 3
RETURN TO THE SOURCE

The ancient tai chi texts exhort students to *return to the Source,* or return to the Tao, through introspection and reversal of the process of creation. This is another reference to the Taoist theory of evolution. Taoists adhere to the idea that for self-discovery one must reverse the path one has followed and discover one's true identity at the Source, understand it, be one with it. Then, using creative evolution with the mind, design a new blueprint for the future. This is a theory of the path to immortality.

The reversal starts with a meditation on your present day situation described as a "full cup of tea." Empty the cup to become pure Yin, devoid of ego, still, silent, ready to accept the knowledge that will fill your empty vessel. The meditative process will take you back to your birth experience or perhaps further, back to the womb. Beyond the womb, you may encounter our energetic connection with animals, and beyond that, eventually reach the Source. In theory, your chi is most pure and powerful at the Source. For this reason, I believe the practice of meditating on the animal forms is of vital importance to those interested in self-defense. Take your mind and chi back in time and swim within the weaving river of energy that flows from the animal kingdom. Drift and bob in its current in order to absorb the pure, supreme, original chi and return with it to the present day.

This is a huge reservoir of pure energy linked to the power of survival. In the grip of a predator, all available chi is used to fend off death. This pure chi, transferred to and stored in the teeth and jaws, fuels the ultimate in survival self-defense as all animals use the teeth and jaws in mortal combat. Those who are able to access this primal chi can expect astounding levels of advancement in their practice of martial arts. This is my discovery.

I question why the masters do not delve into this realm with their students, why such foundational techniques are not part of all core-level instruction. But no matter, I am lifting the veil of mystery, just a bit, so that you may benefit immensely. In short order, the Secret Smile of Laughing Buddha will begin to bring forth many answers to questions concerning the use of teeth and jaws in mortal combat.

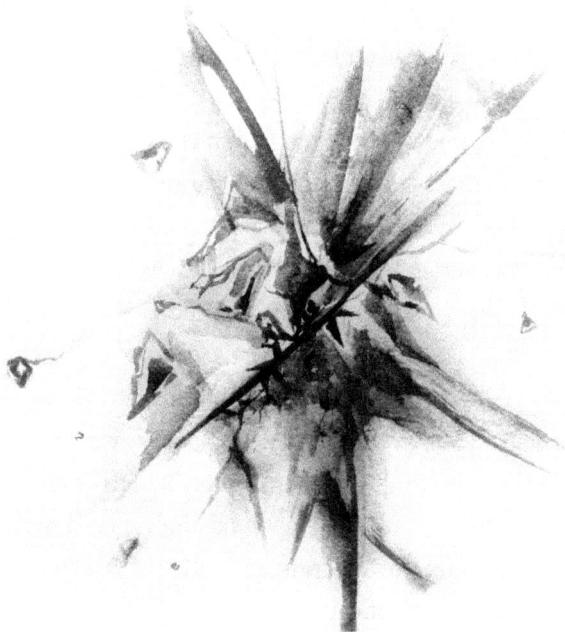

Chapter 4
DIAMOND-STEEL TEETH AND MASSIVE JAWS

For millions of years man depended upon the size and sharpness of his teeth, the bone mass density of the skull and jaws, and the biting force of the jaw muscles when defending himself, and these factors frequently decided the victor in Mortal Combat. Today we have developed superior martial art techniques and weapons of self-defense. Who needs a massive bite force? Such situations are not likely to arise as we drive to work with a double latte in one hand and a smartphone in the other.

However, if one wishes to maintain vibrant health and promote longevity, it is necessary to facilitate the uninterrupted flow of chi. Unfortunately, for many generations the oral cavity has been a blocked and neglected reservoir of original chi, and this holds true in everyday life as well as martial arts development. The average person fails to see the significance of healthy, strong teeth and jaws. People spend little time brushing their teeth in comparison to that devoted to hair styling and fingernail care. And the neglect shown to the oral cavity and surrounding physiology cannot help but have a large, negative effect on overall energy flow. It is highly unlikely that hair might play a major role in protecting your life during combat. And yes, fingernail strength has advantages, but artificial nails have no more value than cosmetic war paint. The teeth, on the other hand... it is easy to imagine the role they might play in a fight to the death.

Here are some recent discoveries that you may find interesting:

Hexagonal Diamond

Diamond is currently regarded as the hardest known material on the planet. But by considering large compressive pressures under indenters, scientists have calculated that a material called wurtzite boron nitride (w-BN) has an even greater indentation strength than diamond. And scientists have also discovered that another material, lonsdaleite—also called hexagonal diamond, because it is made of carbon and is similar to diamond—is even stronger than w-BN and fifty-eight percent stronger than diamond.

Predator X

This fifty-foot long monster is a newly discovered species of pliosaur, and researchers say the reptile ruled the Jurassic seas about one hundred and fifty million years ago. Its anatomy, physiology, and cunning all indicate that it was the ultimate predator, the most dangerous creature to stalk the deep. The forty-five ton creature propelled itself with its four flippers and relied on its crushing jaw power to take out its prey consisting of marine reptiles and fish. Predator X possessed a skull ten feet in length and a bite four times as powerful as that of T-Rex. Researchers estimate that it had 33,000 pounds per square inch (psi) of bite force. (It is interesting to note that the compressive strength of the human tooth is about 30,000 psi.) Bite estimates predict it could crush even the largest four-ton SUV.

Vegetarian Spider

Until recently, all spiders were thought to be carnivorous. A new study reveals that a vegetarian tropical jumping spider has been identified out of some forty thousand meat-eating spider species.

In the late 1800's, naturalists discovered a spider they believed to be carnivorous, but they were uncertain of its exact diet. Biologists studying the spider recently found that it eats the nutrient-rich buds of acacia plants. Also unique to this species is the manner in which it jumps from thorn to thorn in order to escape aggressive ants that live inside the hollow thorns. The spider does occasionally snack on the ant larvae, but the bulk of its diet is plants.

I included these three items because they remind us of how little we truly know, and how much we have yet to learn, of ancient history and the natural world around us. Scientists often make assumptions based on limited data that are later proven to be totally incorrect. It is in this light then that I find it easier to accept the thegotic theory stating that early man consciously sharpened his teeth. Compared to modern man, he would certainly have possessed bone-crushingly sharp teeth and jaw strength. Martial arts masters recognize that ancient man was more in touch with his primordial energy and must have kept it honed for survival. I feel certain that the chi force in primitive man's teeth and bite was incredibly superior to that of 21st century man.

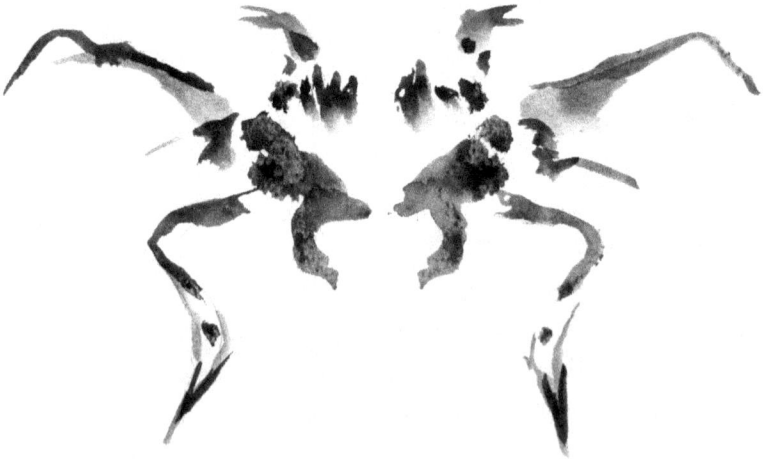

Chapter 5
HUMAN BITE FORCE POTENTIAL

Let's now focus on matters relating to human bite force.

A large dog can exert a bite force of up to 450 pounds per square inch.

A lion can exert a bite force up to about 1000 pounds psi.

An alligator can exert a bite force of 2000–3000 pounds psi.

The human bite force ranges from 55–280 lbs. psi—averaging 162 lbs. psi—and in some cases reaches a maximum of over 970 lbs. psi.

There is an important distinction between bite 'force' and 'pressure.' Human bite pressure has been measured at 5600 psi. However, the compressive strength, or shattering point, of a typical healthy human tooth is up to 30,000 psi. This raises an interesting question: Why do human teeth require a compressive strength of 30,000 psi if man can only produce 5600 psi of bite pressure? Is it possible that primitive man had much greater bite pressure than modern man? Did modern man lose much of his inherent strength because of changes in lifestyle? If the answer is yes, is it possible to regain our original strength, which should logically be much greater due to the 30,000 psi compressive limits of the tooth?

If it were possible to test ancient man's bite force strength and compare it to the force of today's population of relative dental cripples, the cave man would likely win. Every time a dentist drills a tooth, the result is microscopic internal stress fractures that severely weaken resistance to compression and slowly cripple it.

When a lame tooth is challenged with extreme pressure, the biter may either "give up" due to pressure sensitivity or the tooth will shatter. Take special note that a weak tooth—such as one with a large filling, internal crack, or root canal—will suffer a large loss of resistance to compressive forces and easily shatter. Ancient man rarely had serious tooth decay and so would have had no need for dental intervention. His teeth would have had more resistance to breaking and shattering than modern man's compromised tooth structure.

A tooth with an unfilled small cavity will resist compressive forces better than a tooth with a small cavity filled with mercury-silver filling. Studies indicate that a tooth with today's newer bonded white filling is more resistant to dangerous compressive forces than a tooth filled with mercury-silver. If one is undecided about the dangers of utilizing mercury-silver fillings, then this clear advantage of bonded plastic-glass over mercury-silver might be enough to tip the scales.

Twenty-first century tooth filling technology might, in some ways, give our bite force a slight advantage over that of one of our ancestors who had a small tooth cavity. Nonetheless, the person with cavities is sure to have a weaker overall body constitution than one who is free of tooth decay. This has been proven time and again, and was ably demonstrated in the past by the method of examining the teeth in order to ascertain which slaves possessed the hardier constitutions.

There is no denying the fact that mankind today, in general, is weaker in all physical aspects—including teeth and bite strength—compared to ancient populations. Recent findings have almost conclusively proven that primitive man was, by far, physically superior to modern man. Anthropologist John Mehaffey has discovered fossilized aboriginal footprints of six men chasing prey over soft muddy terrain. An analysis showed they reached speeds of twenty-three miles per hour. Today, the world's fastest man can achieve twenty-six mph. But it is highly likely that if the aboriginal men were placed on a hard, flat track and fitted with spiked running shoes, they would easily beat the current world record time. The most accurate measure of the difference in strength and ability between a cave man and a modern athlete would entail a comparison of hunting and combat skills. I would place my money on the caveman.

Other examples of physical superiority from the past: Neanderthal women had ten percent more bulk muscle than modern man. Athens employed rowers who could surpass the achievements of modern oarsmen. Roman legions marched a distance equivalent to one and a half marathons every day while carrying equipment heavier than their body weight. Photographs from the early twentieth century showed young tribal African men accomplishing standing high jumps of up to eight feet as a rite of passage.

And from a mental perspective, as martial artists, our skills and strengths are to a large extent determined by how well we can concentrate and focus our chi. There is no comparison between the shortened attention span and scattered thought processes of modern man and the intensely focused "survivalist" mind of prehistoric man. Concentration and survival are necessarily inseparable. We believe ourselves to be more intelligent, but are we really? Perhaps it is only the vast pool of past experience we have to draw upon to synthesize new data that allows us to feel more intelligent.

But our bite force is unquestionably weaker. When was the last time any of us had to crack open nuts, or crush the neck or leg of a small game animal with our teeth to access the nutritious marrow? It is just not necessary, and one of the results of our softer lifestyle is the neglect of the chi container that comprises the teeth and jaws.

If we can only begin to develop and focus the chi in our mouths to the level of our forebears, and merge this energy into the flow of our major meridians, our capacity for fighting might be restored to the magnificence that nature originally intended.

This is what I have seen in my own personal experience and why I am sharing this information that is RARELY discussed.

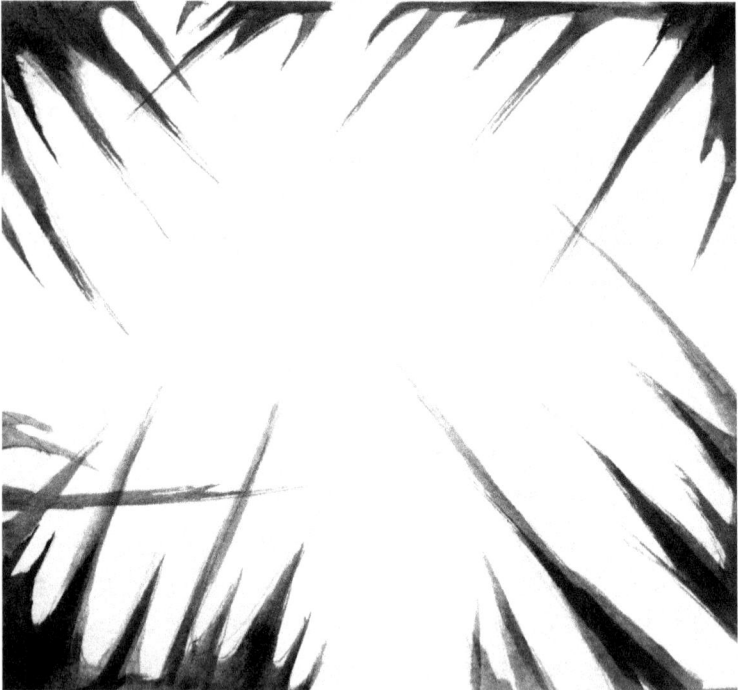

Chapter 6
BITING IN SPORTS

We know that human biting is sometimes involved in violent crimes. The average law abiding citizen, however, also occasionally unleashes the instinct to bite while actively engaged in sports. And athletes functioning at peak intensity often discard all social conformity in order to tap the deep, basic energy needed for victory. The following true events illustrate this point:

Conrad Dobler, the offensive lineman billed as "Pro Football's Dirtiest Player" on the cover of Sports Illustrated in the summer of 1977, admitted to biting Minnesota Vikings defensive tackle Doug Sutherland on the finger.

Ottawa Senators forward Jarkko Ruutu was suspended by the National Hockey League for biting an opponent during a game. Ruutu bit Buffalo Sabres enforcer Andrew Peters on his thumb. Ruutu clamped down on Peters' right glove, catching his teeth on the player's thumb, which is not padded. The force of Ruutu's bite broke the skin and drew blood. As Peters pulled away in pain, his glove was ripped off by Ruutu's bite.

Nashville Predators forward Jordin Tootoo, the pride of Nunavut, was alleged to have bitten the pinkie finger of Columbus Blue Jackets forward Tyler Wright during a game in January 2004.

A high school wrestling coach in Pennsylvania resigned after he allegedly bit one of his wrestlers in the leg during practice.

Former Sydney Swans player Peter Filandia was suspended for 10 matches after pleading guilty to biting an opponent's testicles during a game.

Hockey star Marc Savard was suspended for one game in 2003 when, playing for Atlanta, he bit Darcy Tucker on the glove in a game against Toronto.

New Jersey Devils forward Travis Zajac was wrestling Philadelphia Flyers defenseman Derian Hatcher after the whistle. Zajac offered a face washing to his opponent, and ended up with a bitten middle finger that required stitches.

In 2001, Sevilla midfielder Francisco Gallardo helped teammate Jose Antonio Reyes celebrate a goal by bending down and biting his penis.

In the last fifty seconds of their middleweight bout, with Adrian Dodson five rounds ahead of Alain Bonnamie on the referee's scorecard, the fighters tangled on the ropes and Bonnamie emerged with bite marks to his midriff. Dodson was immediately disqualified.

Rangers center Brandon Dubinsky required a tetanus shot after being bitten on the arm by Caps defenseman Shaone Morrison during an altercation.

And finally, the bite heard 'round the world: Mike Tyson's second fight against Evander Holyfield was stopped when Tyson bit Holyfield's ear in the third round. In a clinch with Holyfield, Tyson tore into his opponent's right ear and bit off a one inch piece of upper ear cartilage and then spit it out as the crowd was just beginning to register the shock. Tyson was penalized two points and the fight continued until he then bit Holyfield's left ear. Tyson was immediately disqualified for biting both ears. His boxing license was later revoked for this and other bad behavior. Kevin McBride, who had fought Tyson four years earlier, told one British tabloid following the famous bout with Holyfield: "Tyson is still crazy. He bit my nipple! I didn't realize it at first, but he had his teeth around it."

And here are a couple of related incidents that were not strictly sports-related:

Elizabeth Loveday was heard shouting "I'll kill you" at her ex-husband while leaving the courthouse. She then took a swing at the court-ordered marriage mediator and bit the woman on the forearm.

Investigators said a Mr. Daniel Allen, an HIV-positive resident of Clinton Township, Michigan, confiscated a football that landed on his lawn while area children and teens were playing nearby and refused to return it to the group. Winfred Fernandis, Jr. approached Allen and asked for the ball. "The suspect (Allen) went nose to nose with the victim (Fernandis) and then bit him on the mouth," said the Detective Captain. "The bite went nearly all the way through his mouth."

But in my opinion, the epic combat bite of all time occurred when David slung a stone into Goliath's eye. Then David, crouching at Goliath's giant ankle, lunged teeth first into his Achilles tendon, chomped down, and dropped Goliath like a cut tree.

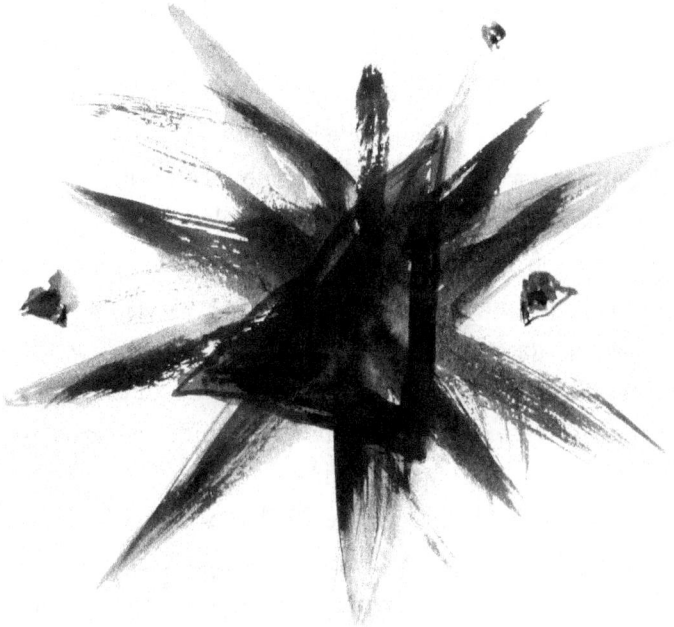

Chapter 7
ALL ABOUT TABOOS

The Physical and Psychological Science
Behind a Lethal Bite

Modern man's teeth are not shaped for puncturing, slashing, and deep penetration of tissue. Today a human bite to the throat would not likely sever any primary blood vessels, but the *pressure* of a strong bite could certainly crush the trachea and tear a blood vessel, leading to a quick death from internal bleeding and suffocation within minutes. (Death from a lethal bite to the neck in an animal usually occurs within five to ten minutes if the carotid artery or jugular vein is severed. Rapid blood loss leads to brain death.) Most martial artists today do not focus on developing the jaw and would have trouble using their teeth to put down an adversary. But in the event that they were relatively successful, the searing wound would put their opponent at a significant disadvantage and end in a slow decline in life force.

Primitive man had a much stronger bite. A deep, pressing bite to the front or side of the neck could easily cause shock, bleeding, suffocation, and paralysis leading to the death of the victim. And in ancient times the bite forces were even greater when we consider the closer connection man had to his energy. It is Intention and Chi that generate power, and during an encounter the first man to engage the throat of the other with such force would certainly be in a winning position.

Today, although the average bite of a human only ranges from 165 pounds up to 285 pounds per square inch, there have been some instances of human bite forces measured in the neighborhood of 1000 pounds per square inch. These modern fellows are much weaker than primitive cave men, so one can only imagine what tremendous bite forces ancient man achieved. A lion is capable of exerting 950 pounds of force; imagine being bitten in the throat by an opponent exploding with a lion's roar!

The anatomy of the throat and neck presents a study in contrasts. The relatively soft throat is very vulnerable to attack as a powerful bite in this area can crush the trachea (windpipe) resulting in rapid death by suffocation. The larynx (voice box) is safer as it rests too high up to be crushed by a human bite. (Primitive man had a hairy throat, which some investigators believe was useful for intimidating predators.) On the neck, the hard posterior of the cervical spine is a combination of skin, fat, fascia, muscle, tendon, ligament, bone, cartilage, blood vessels, and nerves which form a protective padding. Ancient man's short, thick, stocky, hairy neck lent further protection against human bites. It is very unlikely that a bite attack would have occurred from the rear into the cervical spine.

In a fight to the death, every weapon at hand is used. Primitive man, being free from taboos, would have certainly engaged his mighty jaws to bring down an enemy. Then, had the opening presented itself, fingers, toes, and ears would have been open to dismemberment. He would have torn at the flesh with his capable teeth to maul, maim, and rip blood vessels, eventually crushing the windpipe.

However, it is not possible to consider biting as an uncommon occurrence. Those of us with children are aware that they go through a period of imprinting their bite on other children's arms and legs. So common is this developmental behavior in children, a Google search of "child biting" displays nearly 30,000,000 possible hits. But if biting another person is such a natural part of human consciousness and behavior, why should society restrict its use with taboos?

Perhaps because when teeth are used as weapons, vicious passions are involved—those of anger, control, and destruction. One of the most notorious serial killers of the twentieth century, Ted Bundy, savagely bit his victims. During sexual attacks, women are usually bitten on the breasts, buttocks, and legs and men are primarily bitten on the arms and shoulders. These attacks are perpetrated by mentally unstable people, possessed of twisted and distorted energy.

It is easy to see in this light why taboos on biting might have arisen to prevent such aberrant behavior. But when such savagery was unleashed in self-defense against wild animals, the emotional circumstances were far different and the act of biting easily justified.

Exercise to Escape the Taboo on Biting in Self-Defense

There are reasons why few martial art teachers focus on the bite:

First, there are social taboos which can lead to scandal, loss of reputation, and bankruptcy if disregarded.

Second, as a weapon, there is too much deadly power packed into such a small part of the body. Very few students are emotionally ready to approach the study. Mistakes during training might result in serious physical and emotional consequences, and Masters today do not want to take on the liability involved in teaching these techniques.

Third, human nature is such that once one possesses such knowledge and power, there is a reluctance to share it. Masters keep most of these abilities close to the vest as it adds to their allure as an instructor and ensures a healthy income.

Clearly, if one wants to attain the highest levels in the martial arts, teeth and jaw development should be an important part of the training. And this training is not focused only on the physical aspects of teeth, muscle and bone, but rather strengthening the chi of the head, neck and oral cavity.

The following exercise is the first step in breaking the bondage of societal taboos:

1. *Begin in the horse stance. Imagine that you have no arms, or clasp your hands behind your back.*

2. *Imagine you are an animal in a tug of war using your teeth. The head and neck are active while the legs remain rooted. Maintain a Zygomatic Smile. (A zygomatic (Duchenne) smile is the real thing, a genuine heartfelt smile that involves upturned corners of the mouth and wrinkling at the eyes. The brows lower and the eyes seem smaller as the muscles around the eyes contract; it is very difficult to fake or produce on demand.) If you have difficulty visualizing two lions tearing apart a carcass, see yourself as a domesticated dog playing tug-of-war with another dog for possession of a toy.*

3. *When you get a good feeling for the tug, begin taking steps in various directions as the tugging becomes more active.*

4. *At this point, 'grow' back your arms and drop into your usual martial art form in a slow, meditative way, while continuing the tug of war. This can be difficult initially as you have to split your mind. Tai Chi teachers say the eyes lead the hands. (But if you are blind, then what?) In this case the teeth lead the hands. Wherever the teeth lead, the hands should follow, like a whip. I believe putting the whipstock between the teeth is a faster way to learn to connect movement with intention.*

This chi-development exercise is very active, every muscle fiber in the body is cut and tensed, as if in a struggle for survival.

This is not relaxed, sleepy, and dreamlike. You are not here to be hypnotized—this is Fierce Hoopla!

Imagination combined with physical movement will help develop the chi until it feels substantial in the mouth, head, and neck area. After a period of practice, flip into quiet breathing, swallowing, spitting, and vocalization techniques. Connect the oral flow of streaming chi to the great energy channels in the torso. Finally, this approach will make it easier to learn to swim in the Yin-Yang ocean of life.

What you have just read is suckling milk to whet your appetite. If you really want the meat, you need a Master to pre-chew the food and then transfer it to you. Without the Master's extraordinary enzymes, nature's banquet might be hard to digest.

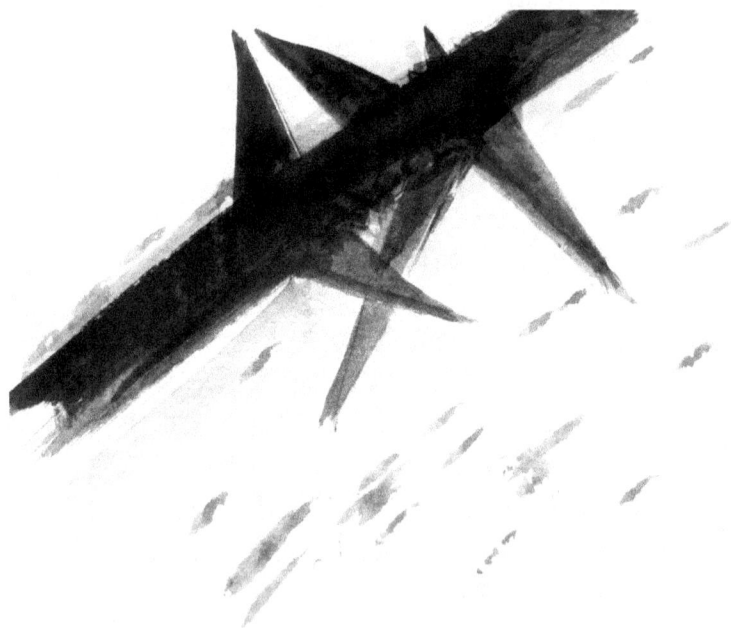

CHAPTER 8
ANATOMY OF A SMILE AND BITE

The zygomatic smile utilizes many more facial muscles than we can easily control voluntarily. It is therefore almost impossible to fake the zygomatic smile, and most of us can immediately distinguish it from a "phony" smile. The Buddha image has been painted, engraved, and sculpted into artwork worldwide and some versions have Buddha displaying a typical zygomatic smile. This representation is known as the Jolly Laughing Buddha. In fact, some depictions show Buddha with a smile so extreme that the eyes and brows are contracted to the point where he looks *fierce*. The artist who first depicted Buddha with a fierce smile understood the qualities of a zygomatic smile. A fierce smile is what I believe to be the martial artist's perfect expression of his art. I call this *"Fierce Hoopla!"*

How are the teeth and tongue positioned during a zygomatic smile? Hearty laughter is usually vocalized with the lungs and larynx, but a hearty smile can be silent. During a silent zygomatic smile, the tongue is pressed against the roof of the mouth, the lower mandible is retruded into anatomic centric relation, muscles of mastication are activated, salivary glands secrete and the ears might even wiggle.

But there is one very important aspect of this smile that is crucial for martial artists: The inward and outward appearance of a zygomatic smile is very similar, *if not identical,* to the visual markers for the head, neck, face, teeth, tongue, and jaws during Mortal Combat. The main difference is that opposite emotions are involved. One is rooted in the joy of laughter and the other springs from savage and aggressive intent. (When you practice driving chi into your teeth and jaws, you will know you are on the right track if you express and feel the identifying markers of a zygomatic smile.)

Studies have found that men who have high testosterone levels with high levels of testosterone tend to smile less. High levels of testosterone are associated with energy, dominance, persistence, combativeness, and focused attention, all qualities that are useful in the martial arts. According to the ancient texts, however, the warrior must be in balance with his environment. So those in harmony—even men with high levels of testosterone—should find ample opportunity to flash a zygomatic smile.

Entering the zygomatic smile state will puzzle one's opponents and give one a psychological advantage. Facing an adversary with a wild facial expression that may be construed either as joy or savagery is quite disarming. This is the same confusion people experience when gazing at the Mona Lisa. Depending on where one stands when studying the portrait, Mona Lisa can appear radiant and serene from one angle and serious from another.

Scientists studied dynamic facial expressions and discovered that our eyes send mixed signals to the brain about smiles. Different cells in the retina transmit different categories of information, or "channels", to the brain. Sometimes one channel is predominant and one sees the pleasant smile, and other times that channel is overridden by another and one's perception is of a grim, determined visage.

Scientists know that the retinal cells which process dead-center vision convey information about facial expressions just as well as the cells that contribute to peripheral vision. Random noise in the path from retina to visual cortex determines whether we see a smile or not. In someone regarding a smile with dead-center vision, the retinal cells might transmit data about the smile that can be interpreted as joyful. When gazing with peripheral vision, the same smile may appear fierce. The end result is confusion, or "Fierce Hoopla," a warrior's most effective weapon.

5 Major Muscles Involved in a Zygomatic Smile

1.) *Zygomaticus major and minor.* These bilateral muscles pull up the corners of the mouth. Total number of muscles: **4**.
2.) *Orbicularis oculi.* One of these muscles encircles each eye and causes 'crinkling.' Total: **2**.
3.) *Levator labii superioris.* Pulls up corner of lip and nose. Bilateral. Total: **2**.
4.) *Levator anguli oris.* Also helps elevate angle of mouth. Bilateral. Total: **2**.
5.) *Risorius.* Pulls corner of mouth to the side. Bilateral. Total: **2**.
Grand total needed for zygomatic smiling: **12**.

Complete Set of Facial Muscles

Auricularis anterior (2)
Auricularis posterior (2)
Auricularis superior (2)
Buccinator (2)
Corrugator supercilii (2)
Depressor anguli oris (2)
Depressor labii inferioris (2)
Depressor septi nasi (1)
Frontalis (1)
Levator anguli oris (2)
Levator labii superioris (2)
Levator labii superioris alaeque nasi (2)
Mentalis (1)

Nasalis (2)
Orbicularis oculi (2)
Orbicularis oris (1)
Platysma (1)
Procerus (1)
Risorius (2)
Zygomaticus major (2)
Zygomaticus minor (2)

Muscles of Mastication (Biting and Chewing)

The teeth could not occlude (come together) or disclude (separate) without the five paired muscles of mastication that make it all possible:

1.) The *Temporalis Muscle* is one of three muscles that close the jaw and clench the teeth.

2.) The *Masseter Muscle* is a "power stroke" muscle. Pound for pound, the masseter is the strongest muscle in the body. It therefore makes good sense to depend on the "strongest" muscle in a struggle of life and death. (Hence my premise of the importance of teeth and jaw to martial artists.)

3.) The *Medial Pterygoid Muscle* elevates and orients the mandible laterally during chewing.

4.) The *Lateral Pterygoid Muscle* is an important muscle responsible for drawing the jaw forward when both the right and left muscles are equally active. It also moves the lower jaw from side to side when the right or left lateral pterygoid is active separately.

5.) The *Digastric Muscle* is most responsible for opening the lower jaw.

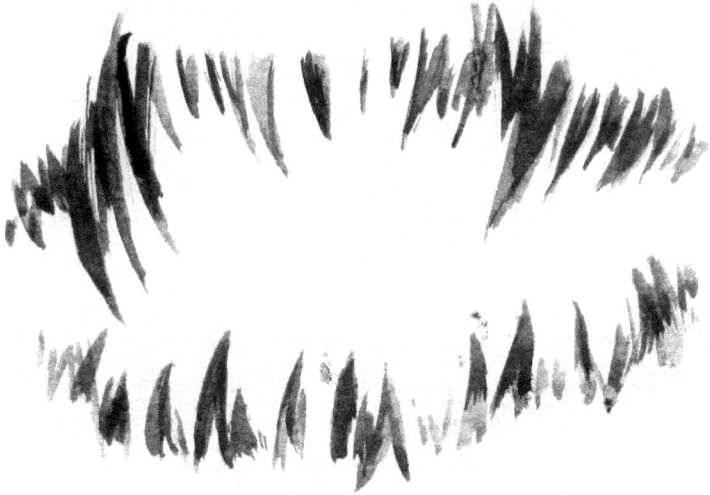

Part Two

"AS YIN AND YANG UNITE, ALL THINGS ARE COMPLETE ON HEAVEN AND ON EARTH."

"The Supremely Profound Principal deeply permeates all species of things but its physical form cannot be seen. It takes nourishment from emptiness and nothingness and derives its life from Nature. It penetrates the past and present and originates the various species. It operates yin and yang and starts the material force in motion. As yin and yang unite, all things are complete on Heaven and on Earth. The sky and sun rotate and the weak and strong interact. They return to their original position and thus the beginning and end are determined. Life and death succeed each other and thus the nature and the destiny are made clear. Looking up, we see the form of the heavens. Looking down, we see the condition of the earth. We examine our nature and understand our destiny. We trace our beginning and see our end.... Therefore the Profound Principle is the perfection of utility."

Yang Hsiung (53 BC–18 AD)

This section examines the Yin and Yang of using the teeth in mortal combat, and all of the chapters are framed in reference to the relation of Yin and Yang. Everything may be broken down into Yin and Yang, and there are two important principles to remember when working with them: There is no such thing as pure Yin or pure Yang; there is always some Yin within Yang and some

Yang within Yin. And each one is always in the process of transforming into the other.

Yin and Yang may be basically viewed in this way:

YANG:

male

active

rising

external

formless

hot, bright

stimulates

firm

YIN:

female

passive

descending

internal

has form

cold, dark

suppresses

yielding

Chapter 9
THE YIN AND YANG OF MUSCLE

In the following chapters I will do my humble best to explain my perception of the Yin/Yang concepts as they relate to the physiology of the face and oral cavity, and also jaw strength, chi, and bite. I feel it is important to understand and be constantly aware of these concepts if one wants to improve their martial arts skills. Let's begin with an examination of two of the strongest muscles in the human body, the masseter and the heart.

In Chinese medical theory, each internal organ is linked with a sensory organ and the heart is connected to another muscular organ, the tongue. There is an energetic pathway between the heart and the tongue, and the tongue is the extension and expression of the heart. People tend to verbalize what is in their heart. Another theory holds that the mind resides in the heart. When one realizes that the tongue, through its connection with the heart, verbalizes and expresses the ideas of the mind, it is easy to see that the harmony between the mind, heart, and tongue constitutes an intimate loving relationship. If disharmony occurs in any of the three, it may be expressed as either excessive talking or complete silence. And when the heart is in harmony, the tongue is able to differentiate different flavors. This is why a person with advancing chronic heart disease usually loses the ability to distinguish flavors in food.

Yang Muscle

The masseter muscle of the jaw is generally considered to be the strongest Yang muscle in the body, and the teeth are seen as the hardest active male energy in the mouth. (The tongue is often

cited as the "strongest muscle in the body," a claim that originated as a metaphor referring to the power of speech. This claim
does not correspond to any conventional definition of physical
strength. However, there may be some truth to this assertion if
one compares the tongue with the masseter, and it is possible to
see the tongue as Yin and the masseter as Yang.)

Yin Muscle

The heart is generally considered to be the strongest Yin muscle in the body, and the tongue, as an energetic extension of the
heart, is the softest active Yin energy in the mouth.

I have discovered that the tongue is actually, in some respects,
stronger than the masseter. When testing the tongue and masseter
in the same space, the tongue is usually dominant. (To my knowledge, there have been no formal experiments wherein the tongue
and masseter have been tested in opposition to each other.) Press
the tip of the tongue with as much strength as is possible against
the roof of the mouth. Then, carefully bite your teeth together as
hard as you can while maintaining maximum pressure with the
tongue.

In my experience, the tongue muscle pressing hard against the
palate seems to prevent the masseter muscle from fully contracting. So in this case the tongue is clearly the stronger of the two
muscles when competing directly against the masseter. But the
tongue will fatigue sooner than the masseter and within perhaps
thirty seconds, the masseter will become dominant and the comparative Yin and Yang qualities of the two will have switched. This
result suggests that the tongue is in need of exercise in order to
increase its aerobic activity. A different result may be obtained by
placing an object between the teeth, in which case the masseter
is dominant.

A. Masseter

The masseter muscle is considered the "power stroke" muscle. It has a high tensile strength in pounds per square inch due to the extreme density of its muscle fibers. Its attachment origin is the inferior part of the zygomatic arch, the protruding bone just below the eye, and it inserts into the inferior part of the ramus of the mandible, or lower part of the arm of the jaw. Its absolute strength, or maximum force exerted, is the greatest of all the skeletal muscles. The muscle attachment to the jaw forms a lever which creates a strong mechanical advantage. It is a very short, dense muscle, and because of its short length, the angle of the lever creates tensile forces greater than any other mechanical (bone-to-bone) lever in the body.

When scientists study and test a particular muscle for strength, they consider three overlapping factors:

- Physiological strength
- Neurological strength
- Mechanical strength

Western science always explains muscle strength in the context of: physiological strength (muscle size, cross sectional area, available cross-bridging, responses to training), neurological strength (the strength of the signal that tells the muscle to contract), and mechanical strength (muscle's force angle on the lever, moment arm length, joint capabilities). Each muscle is isolated and tested against these three factors in a separate container so outside interferences cannot influence the results. If you test two different muscles simultaneously in the same space, one muscle and its testing devices might affect the performance of the other muscle.

Archimedes said, "Give me a long enough lever and the right fulcrum, and I can move the earth." Of course, the power for terrestrial dislocation would have to come from Archimedes' arm, not the lever itself. A more profound definition of strength, in the case of muscles, is that the power to displace the lever begins with the mind and *intention*, which moves the chi through the muscles to the object being displaced by way of the energy meridian pathways, nerve stimulation, and blood flow.

Western science, however, cannot adequately explain 'super human strength' and usually falls back on the explanation of an adrenaline rush as the driving force behind seemingly impossible feats of strength. Adrenaline (epinephrine) is a hormone neurotransmitter, and 'adrenaline rush' refers to the activity of the adrenal gland in a fight-or-flight response when it releases adrenaline causing the muscles to perform fermentation at an increased rate, thereby increasing strength.

The theory of chi better explains the phenomenon of how little old ladies are able to lift an automobile in a split second in order to free a crushed child: adrenaline alone does not offer a convincing explanation.

The General Relativity Theory of Chi states:
Small Muscle + Focused Mind = Relatively *Big Hurt*

B. Heart
There are different aspects of muscle strength:
- *Dynamic strength* = repeated motions
- *Elastic strength* = ability to exert force quickly
- *Strength endurance* = ability to withstand fatigue

The heart is the body's strongest muscle when its strength is calculated as continuous activity without fatigue. It is the muscle that performs the largest quantity of physical work in the course of a lifetime as it work continuously, without pause. One reason this is possible is that the heart is the first organ in the body to be provided oxygen-rich blood after it has left the lungs. As oxygen-rich blood is pumped out of the heart, the majority goes to nourish the body, but some returns immediately into the coronary arteries that supply the heart. This quick return injection provides a more constant supply of highly rich oxygenated blood, and therefore the heart does not have to rely on lactic acid production for energy.

Cardiac muscle is an "involuntary muscle" and found only in the heart. It is very similar to the skeletal muscle of the masseter except in its pattern of fiber arrangement: the masseter has regular, parallel bundles but the heart has irregular, branching angles. The masseter contracts and relaxes in short intense bursts, whereas the heart sustains longer or even near-permanent contractions. Regarding these two muscles from a Yin/Yang, male/female sexual aspect, it is clear that the masseter's male, short, Yang, intense bursts in comparison with the heart's female, Yin, sustained, longer, near-permanent contractions correlate exactly with the art of love-making.

Another variation of the Yin/Yang relationship concerns muscle stimulation. The masseter, and indeed all skeletal muscles, are stimulated externally (Yang) by nerve electrical impulses. The heart cardiac muscle is stimulated internally (Yin) by regularly contracting internal pacemaker cells. All of these muscular descriptions of the heart are Yin in relation to the Yang masseter.

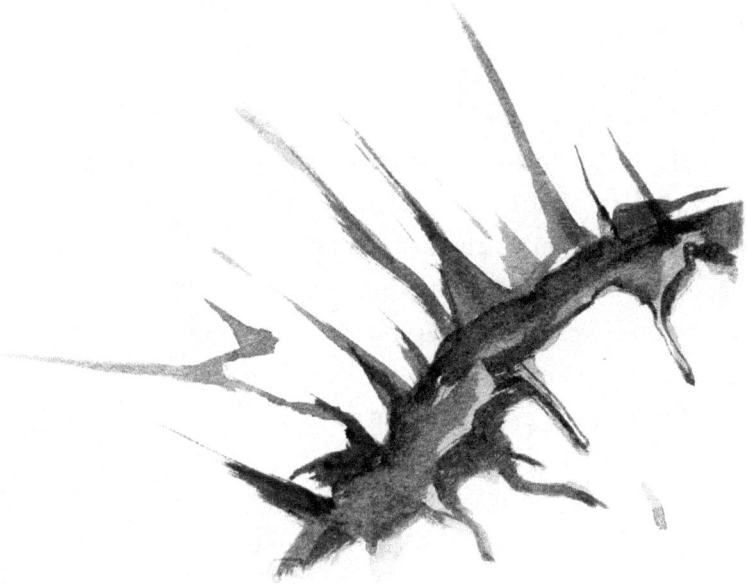

Chapter 10
TONGUE/TEETH

The teeth are the hardest active, male, Yang energy in the mouth and the tongue represents the softest active, female, Yin energy. In this discussion, the teeth and tongue are treated as an example of the interaction of Yin and Yang through the act of mastication (chewing food). The teeth and tongue complement each other: working in concert, they trigger the initial digestive changes in the food that we eat to nourish our bodies.

Teeth and tongue are the Yin and Yang of the masticatory system. A healthy body, mind, and spirit is in balance with all aspects of Yin and Yang. The teeth require the tongue to move and place the food onto the tooth table in order to chew food thoroughly, and the tongue cannot effectively change solid food into a perfect bolus to swallow without the help of the teeth. They must coexist in a complementary and restrictive relationship and harmonize and balance each other.

The teeth protect the tongue by setting up a nearly impenetrable 'fence' around it, and the growth and arrangement of the teeth fall under the tongue's influence. As a child's teeth erupt into the mouth, one by one, the tongue gently guides the 'fence posts' into their appropriate positions. If the child, as an infant, develops abnormal habits with the tongue (e.g. tongue thrust), then teeth develop in the wrong position and at an angle. They may protrude abnormally (buck teeth) and end up in a 'cross-bite', 'end-to-end,' or constricted arrangement.

Yang tooth energy rises. This is seen in the way the teeth erupt, continually growing out of the bone socket until something impedes their movement. The body beautifully arranges this through the development of the upper and lower jaw. The upper jaw teeth grow downward and the lower teeth erupt upward until they meet and stop at just the right time and location, forming a perfect occlusion (bite) for biting, chewing, and speaking. This upward and downward eruption occurs throughout life. When a tooth is extracted, its opposite member will continue to grow and super-erupt abnormally out of its dedicated position, resulting in gum disease, tooth decay, infection, and eventual extraction of the tooth. (This illustrates the importance of the tongue's role in guiding the teeth into their correct position so they form a pristine picket fence without super-eruption.) A perfect tooth arrangement allows easy and thorough mastication of food for the most effective digestion and nutritional absorption.

The tongue consists of sixteen different muscles. It can twist, turn upside down, and bend 180 degrees, and it maintains fitness by exercising itself, pushing against the teeth and upper palate. We swallow two thousand times a day and with each swallow the tongue exercises itself by pushing upward against the palate. However, when a tooth is lost, the tongue no longer has a lateral surface to work against and it begins to lose its muscle tone in the areas where teeth are missing, becoming flaccid and swollen.

The teeth bite and chew food and utilize salivary enzymes to moisten the food into a soft, mushy state. The tongue then forms the mush into a bolus by pushing and rolling it against the upper palate. While the throat prepares to swallow the bolus, the teeth touch together one last time as the tongue goes through a wave-like motion carrying the bolus to the back of the mouth. The final act of the tongue is to pull the prepared food down into the throat where the alimentary canal is waiting to transfer it to the stomach. If the teeth and tongue cannot thoroughly masticate and prepare the food for digestion, the nutrients necessary for optimal functioning of the body will not be effectively assimilated. To a martial artist, the complementary dance between tongue and teeth is vital in a uniquely different manner, as will be shown in later chapters. And of course a well-nourished body is essential for peak performance.

Aside from the nutritive aspect, teeth and tongue also play a major role in the physical act of self-defense. The Yang energy of the teeth can easily be expressed in any number of aggressive and destructive fashions, and the tongue helps support the masseter and other muscles of mastication to provide better biting power. Whether preparing for war or in the heat of battle, a healthy, strong oral cavity is of major import.

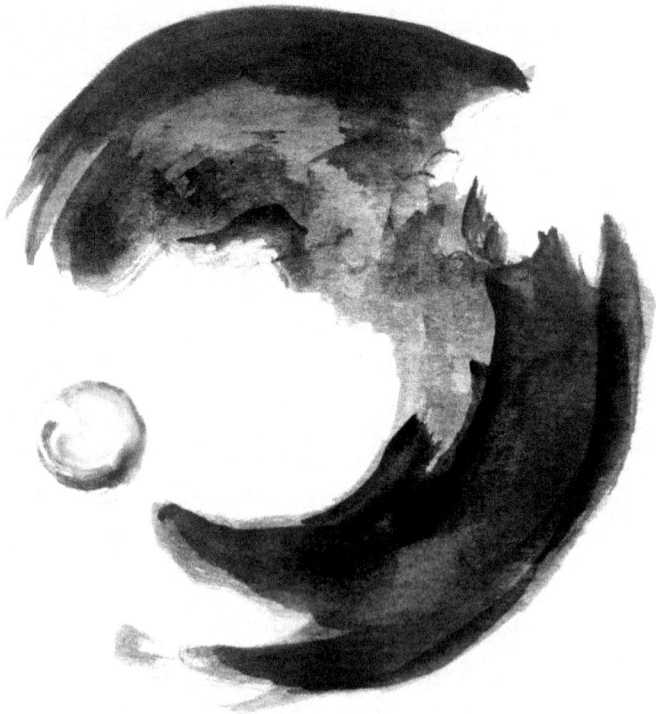

Chapter 11
PASSIVE/ACTIVE

Keeping in mind that one swallows perhaps three thousand times daily, and that with every swallow one touches the tongue to the palate, plus add in all of the speech that takes place, and it's easy to see that the tongue is a very active muscle. The teeth, however, are actually much more active than the tongue. During the waking hours of the day we are constantly tapping, biting, clenching, and grinding our teeth. In the pauses during speech, we find ourselves touching the teeth together. And at night, while we sleep, the action of teeth grinding and tapping continues. The forces exerted during night time grinding can be as great as two hundred pounds per square inch. But during sleep the tongue is passive and recovering from the day's work, even as the teeth continue to "grind through" the events of the day.

The continuous action of tapping, grinding, clenching and biting is medically termed *bruxism*. Nearly everyone in our industrial and technologically advanced countries will suffer from this condition at some time in their life. It is one of the most destructive forces wearing down the teeth, slightly ahead of acid-filled, carbonated soft drink beverages such as colas and energy boosters. Grinding is a subconscious muscle activity and most grinders grind without realizing it. The wake-up call comes when the teeth become sensitive to cold temperatures and/or chewing, one chips a tooth while sleeping or develops facial soreness. Moderate and occasional bruxism is considered necessary to resolve psychological issues that arise from day to day living, but threatens the health of the teeth and jaws if the bruxism becomes chronic, severe, and pathological.

I identify bruxism as a vibration of the teeth due to the bottom teeth rubbing against the top. Because of the hard calcium phosphate mineral structure of teeth, they also vibrate in harmonic frequency with vocal sound waves. Hard structures of the mouth, such as teeth and bone, respond more palpably to sound waves than do the soft tissue and muscle. Sound waves do travel through soft tissue, of course, making possible the medical use of ultrasound diagnostic devices. When the teeth vibrate, however, the intensity will leave no doubt that they are conducting at a greater perceptible frequency than the soft tissue. Excessive vibration initiates a protective mechanism from the tooth pulp, or center of the tooth, where vital fluids and vascular tissue (capillaries and nerves) live. The pulp's primary function is to provide nourishment to the tooth and it is, in most cases, the principle source of pain within the mouth.

As we age, the Yang teeth very clearly change size, shape, and structure. The pulp continuously creates a hard protective dentin shell. This yellow dentin lies just beneath the surface of the white enamel and, in the face of irritants, the pulp accelerates the formation of new calcified dentin as a defense, thickening the hard protective casing around the pulp. With each passing year, chronic irritation and vibration—such as clenching and grinding—thickens the dentin to the point where the pulp begins to shrink in size. Chronic irritation also stimulates the pulp to create calcified "stones" within the pulp chamber.

The Yin tongue, with its taste buds, vascular tissue and nerves, on the other hand, does not change significantly in size and structure as we age. When examining the Yin and Yang qualities of teeth and tongue, it is obvious that the teeth are far more active than the tongue. They constantly vibrate against one another in response to vocal sound frequencies from within the mouth. Environmental vibrations such as automobile traffic, human footsteps, airplane and industrial machine noises, even the quaking crust of the earth, transmit waves through the soles of the feet into the bones of the human skeleton and upward directly into the teeth. Teeth also "jiggle" with the arterial pulse, and the blood pressure from surrounding capillaries constantly pumps and thrusts the tooth in and out of the bone socket. The teeth are clearly more active/Yang than the comparatively passive/Yin tongue.

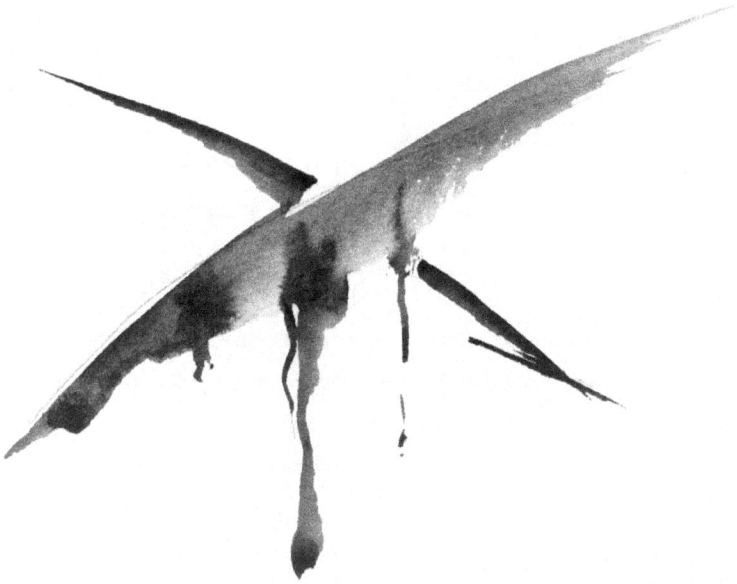

CHAPTER 12
THE YIN AND YANG OF CHEWING AND SWALLOWING

The digestive system is a continuous tube-like structure measuring about forty feet in length from the mouth to the anus that is designed to transport and transform solids and liquids, rendering them suitable for absorption and excretion. The teeth and tongue, together with salivary enzymes, prepare food for digestion by physically grinding it and breaking it down into small pieces to begin the digestive process. The teeth cut and grind the food and the tongue assists in moving it around during chewing and swallowing. During the process, proteins unwind so they can be separated into their component amino acids, thereby breaking the food into molecular pieces that your body can use for nourishment.

The food is then swallowed due to two types of muscle function: the first is voluntary and involves the tongue lifting the food bolus upward and backward until it reaches the back of the throat, at which point all actions become involuntary, meaning that they occur outside of one's conscious control. During the first of a series of involuntary phases, muscles move the food down and back into the esophagus to the point where the food is actively moved through the esophagus to the stomach. This action occurs through coordinated movements by constrictor muscles lining the esophagus and is not the result of gravity.

There is a definite Yin/Yang relationship between the teeth and tongue during the act of chewing and swallowing. The teeth and masseter exert an average force of twenty to thirty pounds psi on the back molars while the tongue pushes upwards against the palate with a force of about four pounds psi. In the process of rendering the food small enough to swallow, the teeth represent the greater Yang force and the tongue may be seen as lesser Yin.

To use an overly simplified analogy, the mouth is grossly similar to a nuclear reactor wherein fission releases energy. Nuclear fission is a nuclear reaction in which a heavy nucleus (Yin) such as uranium splits into two lighter nuclei (Yang), releasing energy as it does. One can say the lighter nuclei rise with the release of energy and rising is a Yang characteristic. It is easy to see the similarities between fission and mastication: the teeth break up the dense food (Yin) into lighter particles that release energy (Yang) during the digestive process. Ideally, mastication should continue until the heavy Yin particles of food are transformed into a Yin fluid ready for transport downward to the stomach. The teeth, therefore, function to release Yang energy from solid food (smaller particles) while transforming the food into a liquid (Yin) component. Conversely, the tongue takes the broken, lighter Yang food particles and passes them downward to the esophagus for their descent into the stomach, thus demonstrating the tongue's descending Yin characteristic.

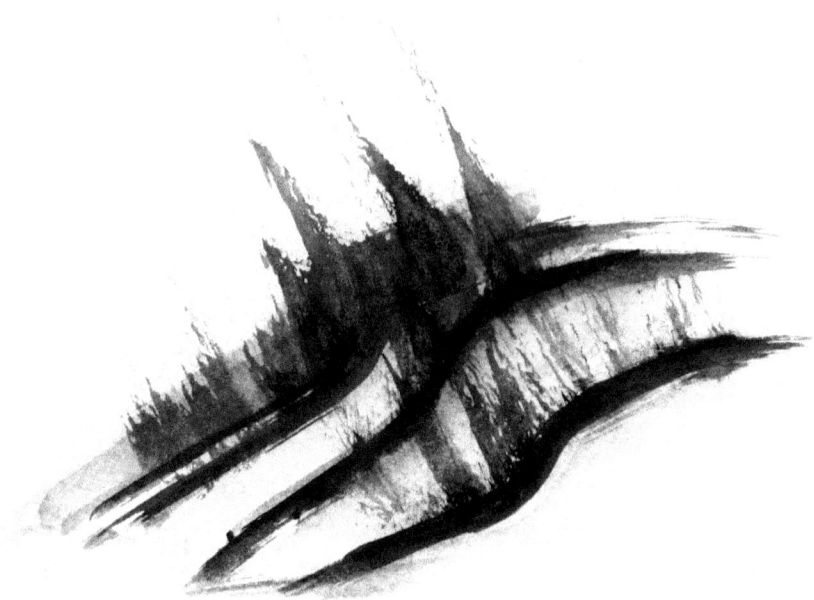

CHAPTER 13
THE INS AND OUTS OF THE GI TRACT AND WHY TWO NATURAL SETS OF TEETH IS NOT ENOUGH

The GI tract, or alimentary canal, is a passageway for food to be transported, absorbed, and released, thereby serving as the body's food processing plant. Thirty to forty feet long from esophagus to anus, it is a muscular, extended, and convoluted tube that is actually connected with the external skin. Digestion begins at the mouth where food is chewed and mixed with saliva, adding moisture containing the enzyme amylase, which is necessary to begin to break down starches. The tongue molds the food into a ball mass known as the bolus. The bolus travels down the esophagus and through the pharynx by a muscular contraction called the peristaltic movement.

Once the bolus enters the stomach, the hormone gastrin arouses the secretion of acidic juices which further aid in the digestion of the food mass. After the stomach carries out its role in the digestive process, the food is no longer in a solid state, but has now been reduced to a liquid called chyme. The chyme travels into the small intestine to the duodenum where most of the digestive process occurs as different enzymes are released by the pancreas and glands in the intestinal wall to disassociate each molecule.

At the end of this process, each complex molecule has been broken down into its simple state. For example, carbohydrates are broken down into simple sugars, proteins into amino acids, and fats into glycerol and fatty acids. These substances are absorbed and utilized for the proper functioning of the human body. Substances that cannot be broken down by the body pass through the large intestine where the last of the water, ions, and salts are reabsorbed and the remaining solid material, called feces, is expelled through the anus.

The teeth and tongue are the gateway into the GI tract. Both arise from embryonic epithelial cells connected to skin cells and, as such, are considered to be "outside" of the body. The tongue, however, is deeper inside (Yin) the canal and the teeth are more external (Yang).

Many of us have learned, thanks to childhood trauma, that teeth avulse, or are torn out, pretty easily. The phrase "harder than pulling teeth" is widely misunderstood by the public. Pulling teeth is actually very simple if the root shape and surrounding bone density does not interfere: young conical roots with thin cortical bone plate actually extract with very little effort, and an elbow or fist to the mouth is more than enough to readily loosen and remove most teeth. The mature tooth is connected to the body by a network of fragile, hair-like periodontal ligaments which tear easily when sufficient lateral force is applied to the tooth, leaving it floating in the bone socket.

The reason for this is that the vertebrate mammal, especially the human, has teeth that have developed as expendable appendages. This expendable nature of teeth is considered a Yang characteristic. The embryo creates a tooth bud from stem cells, which, after flowering into a tooth, will eventually drop from the stem or mandible (jaw bone). The process occurs only twice in most people's lifetimes, resulting in one set of twenty baby teeth and one set of thirty-two adult teeth.

The tongue is a permanent appendage and is therefore regarded as being Yin because of that and due to its more internal relationship to Yang teeth. The anatomy of the tongue makes it impossible to tear away from its deep mounting as it is firmly attached to the body by thick muscle fibers and a vast network of nerves. The body of the tongue is made up of muscles covered by lingual mucous membranes and it is anchored to the floor of the mouth and at the rear by muscles attached to a spiny outgrowth at the base of the skull. More specifically, the muscles are attached to the lower jaw and to the hyoid bone (a small, U-shaped bone which lies deep in the muscles at the back of the tongue) above the larynx.

One major concern regarding teeth is their endurance and how to maintain their health throughout a normal human lifespan. People today in the industrialized nations live on average almost eighty years, or twice the life-span usually associated with our ancestors throughout history. An American at the time of the Revolutionary War could expect to live thirty-five years, and it was rare for people to survive much past that age. George Washington was an exception: he managed to live sixty-seven years, but late in life he required dentures. Most people in that era had poor oral hygiene and also were afflicted with the destructive habit of bruxism, making it almost impossible for teeth to endure past fifty-five years of age. In the modern world, teeth can withstand about forty years of neglect before either falling out or needing to be removed due to disease.

Scientific data seem to indicate that the human body is 'designed' to last for one hundred and fifty years and possibly as long as two hundred and fifty years. I believe human beings are probably capable of expressing a third tooth bud for a third set of teeth that would enable us to masticate well into our third century of life. It does not make sense that Mother Nature would fail to supply us with sufficient teeth to see us through our natural lifetime. Evidence for a natural second set of adult teeth does not exist, but the premise is sound. In my dental practice, I have seen many examples of relatively healthy people ninety years old—and even older—who still sport a full set of hardy, beautiful teeth. Should they remain otherwise healthy, there is no reason that their teeth should not serve them well for another sixty years; I am convinced of this certainty.

According to my theory, a set of healthy, well-formed adult teeth should endure for one hundred and twenty years in a person of otherwise exceptional good health. Accepting the possibility of the existence of a third tooth bud, then that would mathematically allow for the possibility of a two hundred and fifty year human life span: 12 years (baby teeth) + 120 years (1st set of adult teeth) + 120 years (second set of adult teeth) = 252 years total. I have no doubt that we will soon have proof of this theory's validity. We need only discover whether the trigger for a second set of adult teeth has been lost in the human genome or, if it still exists, how to naturally reestablish it.

Non-mammalian vertebrates form teeth repeatedly through a process very similar to the mechanisms humans have for replacing hair. Why do we lack this process in regard to teeth, yet retain it in regard to hair? Scientists searching for the answers to such questions may one day soon be able to grow new teeth by utilizing adult stem cells. But scientific intervention is not necessary according to my theory: if we follow nature's laws for good health, our stem cells will naturally awaken at the proper time to form the tooth buds for a third set of teeth.

Chapter 14
FORM/FORMLESS

A tooth whose congenital and/or permanent external shape is changed through insult or injury, cannot regrow to its original shape. If one chips or breaks a tooth, there is no mechanism within it or the body that will heal and return it to its previous normal and functional state and shape. Scientists are currently developing ways to re-grow human enamel and are able now to regenerate an entirely new tooth. No one at the time of this writing, however, has shown that the tooth can be recreated into an exact reproduction of the original. After serious insult, the energetic memory, or blueprint, of a tooth is lost and I consider it to become formless.

The tip of the tongue, on the other hand, after suffering severe damage can regenerate to its original form. The energetic memory is contained primarily within the intrinsic muscles that actually allow the tongue to regenerate and grow back into its original shape and structure. Unfortunately, if it is damaged too far back in its body, the regenerative properties begin to decrease and it may become unable to fully redevelop. The tongue, therefore, possesses a limited memory blueprint from which it can reproduce itself. The tongue, after serious injury, is considered to retain its form for this reason.

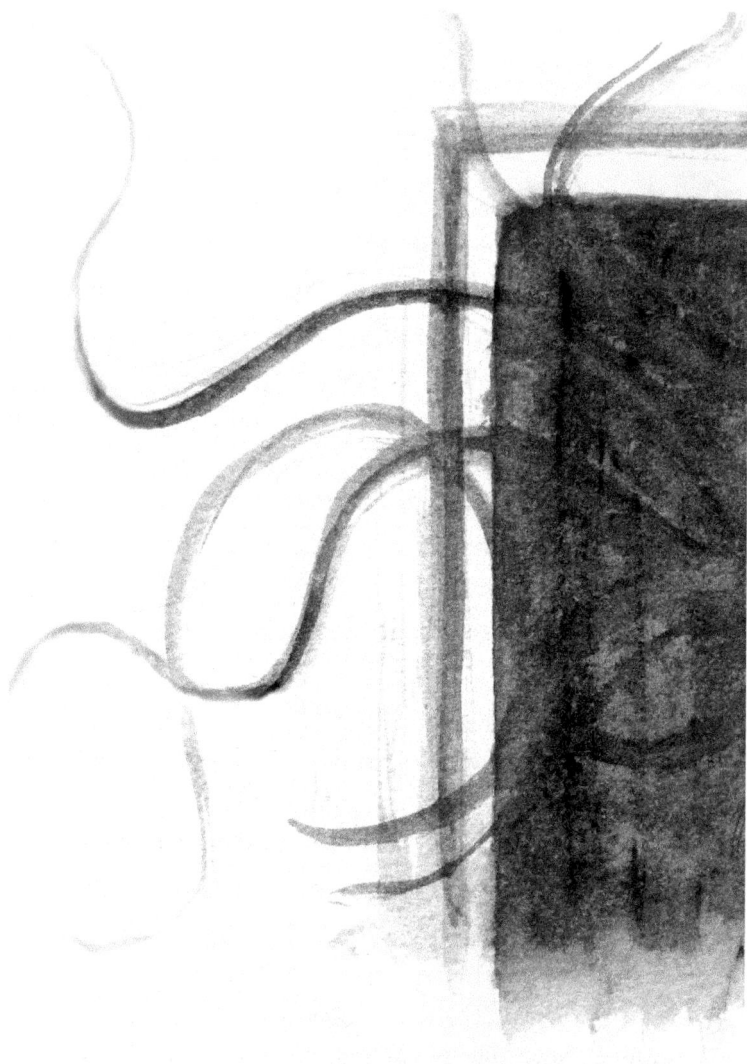

164

Chapter 15
PULP FRICTION

There are two basic components to powerful chewing and biting forces. First, there are the "chompers," or the teeth and muscles—mainly the masseters—used for mastication. The chompers cut, tear, break, grind, and mash the food. And the second component is the tongue, which is in charge of moving the food along the thirty-two tooth arches in order for every bite of food to be thoroughly "chomped." The tongue muscles develop before the masticatory muscles and the tongue's growth is completed by birth. The masticatory muscles develop later and are still not complete at birth. The teeth develop even later: the third molar wisdom tooth crown is completed between twelve and sixteen years of age.

Consider the embryonic stages of growth and see Yang as hot and developing, and Yin as cold and complete or not-developing. The teeth and masseters are seen as Yang/Hot because they continue to develop until the adolescent years, in contrast to the Yin/Cold tongue which ceases developing embryonically by birth.

The walls of the blood vessels within the tooth pulp are of necessity very thin because the pulp is protected by a hard, unyielding sheath of dentin. The dense capillary network just beneath the dentin is known for its rapid blood flow and extremely high blood pressure. Toothaches occur when the swelling pressure of an inflamed pulp has nowhere to expand and release within the constricted encasement of the hard enamel-dentin crown. All of these features constitute a Yang/Hot environment. With age, however, the tooth pulp becomes less cellular and ultimately more fibrous leading to an overall reduction in volume due to the continued deposition of dentin. These natural changes are all signs of aging, or Yang becoming Yin.

The tongue's blood vessels, in comparison, exist within the spacious compartment of the tongue and mouth. Its vasculature does not suffer from heat symptoms as does the compressed pulp. The tongue and its blood vessels are cooler, more Yin and free to move within the mouth, unlike the tooth pulp which remains caged within a hot, enamel-dentin crown. As the body grows older, the tongue remains cooler within its more spacious environment and appears to age less than the teeth, which all constitutes even more evidence that the teeth are Yang/Hot and the tongue is relatively Yin/Cold within the functioning oral cavity.

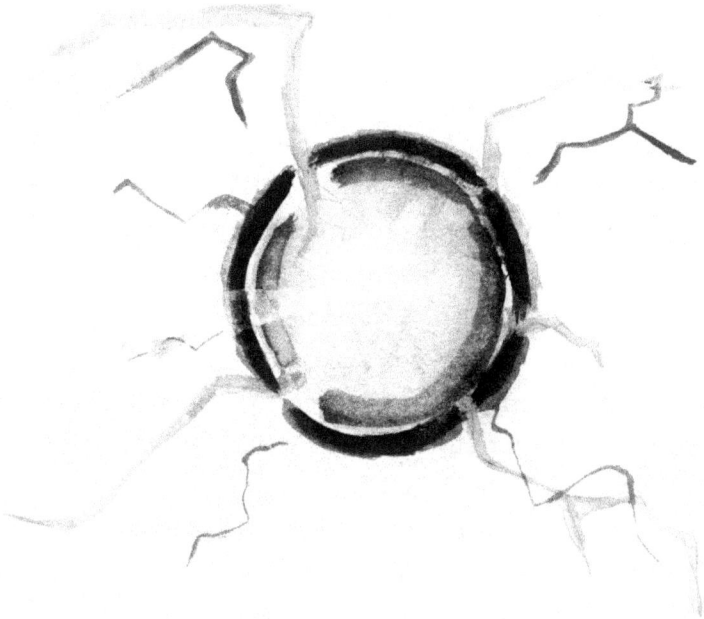

Chapter 16
FIRM/YIELDING

Anyone who has ever accidentally bitten their tongue is intimately familiar with its yielding nature. In less than a millisecond it snaps back away from the offending tooth. Teeth, however, are relatively firm and unyielding in their attachment within the bone socket. A tooth barely senses that it is about to chomp into the soft tongue and it requires a hard bone, seed, or nut shell to send a clear message that there is a problem. And because teeth do not yield in any significant manner, they must therefore send this message to the brain, where it is further relayed to the masseter, to cease the action of biting. The masseter relaxes and then awaits further instructions before contracting again. After generating a few descriptive cuss words and tears, the brain rewires the pathways and allows the masseter to resume chewing.

Teeth literally hang by a threaded mesh of tangled ligaments within bone sockets and do not yield easily without the assistance of the reflex response of the motor units of the five pairs of muscles of mastication. This slight yielding nature of the tooth is mostly dependant upon the immediate inhibition response of the masseter muscle, but the tooth may also yield in a very minimal way through its periodontal attachment to the bone. It is precisely due to the fact that teeth do not readily yield that a high impact force can easily knock one out.

Studies have shown that stimulating the teeth evokes either a facilitating (boosting) or inhibiting (stopping) reflex response in the masseter. A **slow push** on a tooth will result in exciting and facilitating the masseters to contract, while a **brisk tap** on the tooth will elicit a significant reflex inhibition, or cessation of the biting action. Inhibition of the jaw-closing muscles tends to protect the teeth when one bites unexpectedly on a hard object while chewing.

The tongue, however, yields directly to unpleasant forces and does not have to rely on other muscles to protect itself. It is also capable of retracting, which is a yielding, or Yin, action. The tongue plays a valuable role in other yielding actions such as blowing bubbles with bubble gum, and whistling.

Teeth are firm and unyielding and therefore prone to chips, fractures and breaks—all Yang characteristics. The tongue is yielding and Yin.

Part Three

AWAKENING THE BEAST OF FIERCE HOOPLA

Chapter 17
BUDDHA TOOTH

Legend has it that when the Buddha died his body was cremated in a sandalwood pyre and his left canine tooth was retrieved from the funeral pyre by Arahat Khema. A belief grew that whoever possessed the sacred tooth relic had a divine right to rule that land. Today there are at least four separate countries claiming to possess one of Buddha's teeth: according to the Chinese Government, historical texts show that only two relics exist, one held in Beijing and the other in Sri Lanka. Buddhists in India and Singapore, however, also lay claim to Buddha tooth relics. Whether these relics are authentic or not makes for interesting conversation over coffee or tea, but I wonder—what was the original reason that one of Buddha's teeth was held in such reverence?

'Buddha' translates as 'Awakened One', or someone who has awakened from the sleep of ignorance and sees things as they really are. A Buddha is one who is completely free of all faults and mental obstructions. I am not personally enlightened enough in the tenets of Buddhism, or in the details of the life of the Buddha, to discuss these matters in depth. I am curious, however, about one aspect of the many carvings, statues, portraits and other depictions of the Buddha. Why is he sometimes depicted with a large smile, and at other times with no smile? *And what about the teeth behind the smile* that is portrayed in so many images? Interestingly, the first known images of Buddha depicted him without a smile.

The jolly "Laughing Buddha" smile is, without doubt, my favorite, and it is the epitome of a true zygomatic smile. In China, he is known as the Loving, or Friendly, One and is said to have been based on an eccentric Chinese Ch'an (Zen) monk who lived over one thousand years ago. His large protruding stomach and jolly smile have given him the common designation "Laughing Buddha", and he is known as a deity of contentment and abundance. According to legend, if one rubs the Laughing Buddha's great belly, it brings forth wealth, good luck, and prosperity.

All forms of portraits have been long regarded as high art and, at its best and most sublime, portrait painting has been considered with an almost reverential admiration. Historically, the portrait subject patiently endured a two-hour sitting and would not have been inclined to attempt to hold a definite expression of any kind, nor would the painter have thought of making such a request. A serious expression on the face of the subject was typical of fine portraits, and lightness of mood was seldom expressed in portraiture. This constraint led to the tendency for portraits to be composed, restrained, and even dignified. And throughout history, portraits have never depicted the teeth in a smile. The most famous smile, that of the Mona Lisa, is a perfect example.

It was not until the age of photography that teeth became an important component of the smile. Today's standard is a broad, toothy smile, and white teeth are crucial in creating a successful image. Yellow, stained teeth are never found in the portfolios of famous people. And according to recent surveys, yellow teeth are a major turn-off during the act of making love. The portrait smile still remains a point of contention, but the current trend tends toward naturalness and you will see more lighthearted expressions represented today than in the past.

My interest in the visage of saintly figures such as Buddha, Jesus, Muhammad, Zoroaster, and Socrates lies in the deeper core meaning. Are there secrets to be revealed behind the smile/no smile, behind broad, smiling exposed teeth? What is the meaning of teeth hidden behind closed lips? Is there more to explore and understand than what history has written?

So be it. Allow me to plant seeds in your mind that may blossom into food for thought as you journey along your Path.

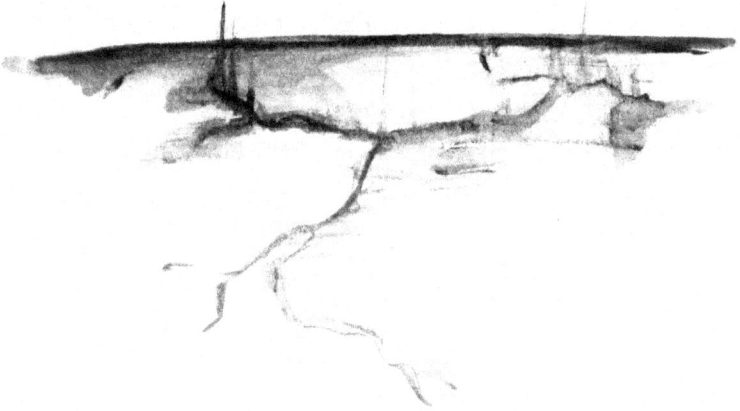

Chapter 18
THE TEETH AND TONGUE
OF LIFE AND DEATH

To study the teeth and tongue, in my opinion, is to study a microcosm of Life and Death. First, let us examine the role of the tongue. All human instinctual drives link with the tongue. Infants use the tongue for drawing nourishment from the mother's breast. Babies use the "tongue reflex," which pushes out any foreign food or substance, to protect against choking before they are old enough to digest solid food. In a manner of speaking, the tongue reflex is the FIRST instinctive self-defense skill a human being uses to preserve its life. In adults, the tongue also plays a part in propagating life: its use in foreplay leads to procreation.

The tongue directs the ideal placement of the erupting teeth within the arches. And after the teeth begin to erupt, the baby is, in effect, taking greater charge of its destiny as the teeth become its second weapon used to defend against real and/or imagined threats. Babies and young children bite vulnerable body parts to gain needed attention and ward off unfamiliar threats in order to preserve life. It is easy to see how teeth give and take life: they masticate and soften food into a liquid state, readying the nutritive potential for digestion, and their bite forces thwart imminent danger to life. But it is the tongue, with its ability to form words that are potentially more devastating than any WMD, that is truly man's ULTIMATE WEAPON.

The teeth and tongue play an important role in balancing the Yin and Yang of the entire body. When the tip of the tongue touches the roof of the mouth, it connects two major energy pathways of the body—the Governing and Conception vessels. And when the teeth of the upper and lower jaws are touching, it contributes secondarily to connecting the two energy channels. The Governing Vessel is the confluence of all the Yang channels, over which it is said to "govern," and it is also known as the "Sea of Yang." This is due to its location and pathway because it flows up the mid-line of the back—a Yang area of the body—and over the top of the head and down to the upper palate. It may be used to increase the Yang energy of the body. The Conception Vessel, or "Sea of Yin," plays a major role in Qi circulation and monitoring and directing all of the Yin channels. It connects with the lower palate, and by joining the two channels with tongue and teeth in the oral cavity, Yin and Yang may be balanced throughout the body.

The teeth and tongue have a beautiful, symbiotic relationship: the tongue gently rubs, cleanses, and massages the teeth, and the teeth—the hardest substance in the body—create an almost impenetrable barrier protecting the tongue. Each supports the other, and neither can fully exist without its complement. Nature designed the teeth and tongue to last a lifetime. In the case of teeth, at least three sets are needed to serve the body until the age of two hundred and fifty years is reached. The tongue never wears out. Through knowledge of the tooth and tongue, life and death become more meaningful.

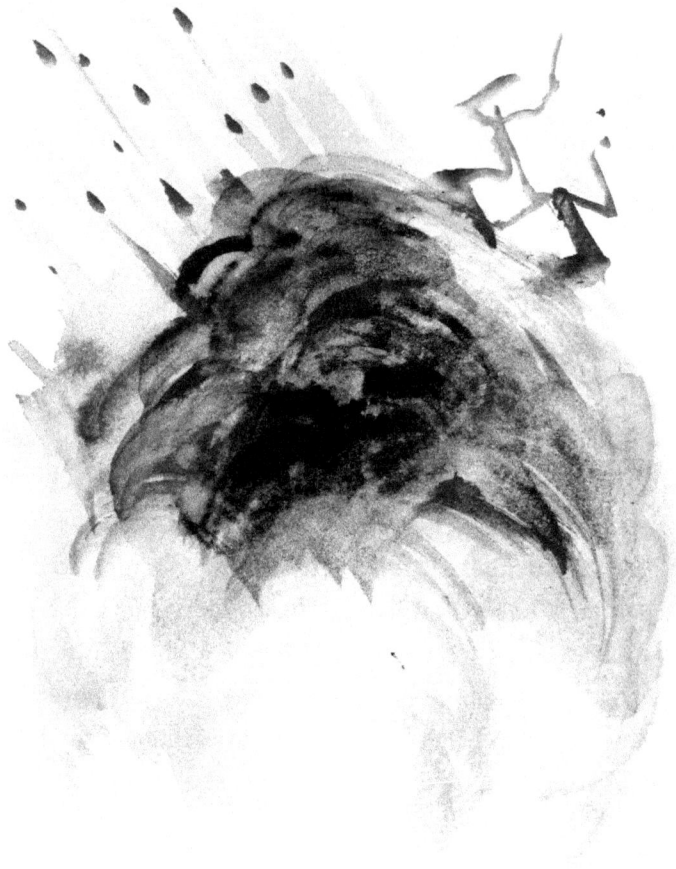

Chapter 19
THE MISSING LINK

Anthropologists searching for the missing link to our original ancestor discovered an ape skeleton in Ethiopia in 1994. This revolutionary finding reinforces the theory that chimps and humans evolved separately from a common ancestor. Our oldest known human ancestor to date, named 'Ardi' by her discoverers, roamed the forests of Africa over four million years ago. She was short, hairy, and had long arms and—similar to today's humans—stubby upper canine teeth. This is significant because scientists previously believed that our common ancestor would prove to be more chimp-like—and chimps possess long, sharp canine teeth.

The assumption exists that because Ardi's canine teeth are smaller than those in chimps and apes, this hominid species did not use them to fight and compete for mates. I believe a vital piece of information was left out of the reasoning that led to that conclusion, and the missing link in this string of logic is chi. Anthropologists are not knowledgeable about human energy and I feel that this shortcoming has led to a misrepresentation of the relics. Just because Ardi's canine teeth are not as long and sharp as those of chimps should have NO bearing on their use for fighting and competing for mates.

Contrary to popular belief, size and shape is not everything and I do not believe that a stubbier canine tooth is less effective in mortal combat than a long sharp one, or that the longer, sharper version guarantees success. Every variety of tooth shape and size possesses Chi Potential. Combatants must necessarily utilize all of their tools—without focusing on any perceived disadvantages or advantages—to the fullest extent in order to triumph. And the focus should be on how to bring out the full potential of the teeth by refining the chi. Believe me, if teeth are possessed of refined chi to the extent that they can bite through iron, the shape and size are irrelevant. The person who can develop and use their chi will ultimately win the fight over another who relies only on the physical.

At this juncture of my dissertation, it is time to focus on biting during mortal combat. This chapter is the missing link for the development of chi in the jaw muscles, bones, and teeth. All that has come before—from the Buddha's smile, Yin-Yang properties, Ardi, Predator-X, to disagreements about the importance of size and function—merely constitutes a simply chewed meal, the relevance of which is to illuminate the possibility of something beyond the obvious. But when the goal is developing martial arts skills, one must bite hard and deep into the hide.

In order to take another step forward in your understanding of energy within the martial arts, focus on the teeth and tongue. Every part of the body connects to and benefits the whole, and the teeth and tongue are no less important than the foot and fist when in combat. They may, however, be a missing link in your quest to understand chi and chi potential. It is necessary to use imagination, visualization, and a deep understanding of your inner feelings in order to discover what lies behind the Laughing Buddha Smile. At all times, remember, "Dance with Fierce Hoopla!"

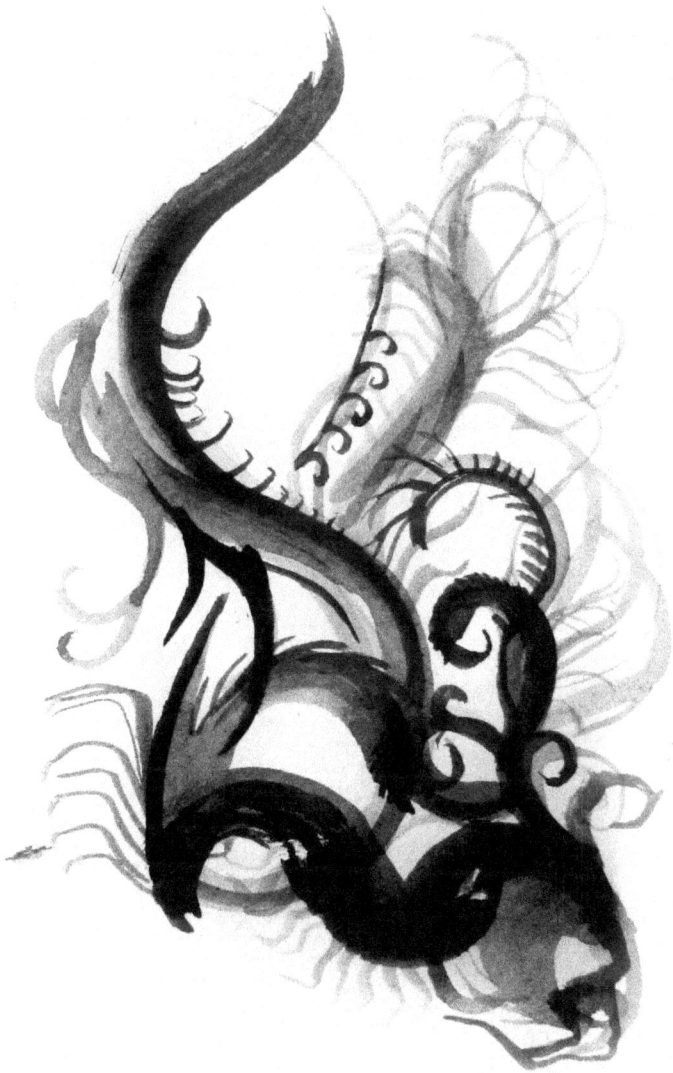

PART FOUR

LIGHTNING AND THUNDER

Chapter 20
FEEL THE VICTORY

American football players may be taught to "bite the football." This is a tackling technique taught from day one to the youngest of players. Unless a tackle is properly and safely executed, there is imminent danger of concussion/mild traumatic brain injury or cervical vertebral fracture with resulting paralysis, and the technique of "biting the football" prevents the player from spearing his opponent with the helmet during a tackle. Players are instructed to keep their eyes on the football, or the player being tackled, at all times. The head should be up, but to the side of the player being tackled so that at the moment of contact it is possible to imagine biting the football. When a tackle is performed correctly, the tackle should be with the shoulder, not the face or helmet.

In order to take this training a step beyond the physical and into the world of chi, one must practice in a quiet setting. The intensity of hard physical tackles and competition is a distraction from chi nurturing and development. Once the practice of utilizing the chi has been mastered, it is then possible to incorporate this technique into the physical aspect of tackling. When one practices biting the football 'energetically,' an elevated amplitude of energy that will explode on contact is developed and tackles have more grace and "pop" than if reliance is on the physical body alone. Consciously exercising chi potential when tackling will also develop an Energetic Protective Shield around the head and neck.

Biting the football is a good introduction to the exploration of the practical use of teeth during mortal combat. The principle and training is the same: the goal is to drive and guide one's chi into the head, neck, face, mouth, teeth, jawbone, gums, and tongue. Once the chi that is being directed into these areas is sensed, or felt, begin pumping the chi like air into a tire to increase the pressure. (This is not the time or place to discuss the benefits of pumping chi into the teeth. Discussing the multiple benefits might plant suggestions, and it is better for the individual to experience and witness their own rewards.)

When I do this practice, I use imagination to take myself to the time of Ardi, and even beyond, to our unknown common ancestor. Simply biting a football in my present surroundings does not allow me to truly experience this technique. I visualize myself as primitive and naked, hair covering my body, hunting for food with my eyes wide open and all six senses fully alert! The hunted animal appears and suddenly I'm fighting—life and limb, tooth and nail—for my next meal. Muscles cut and flex, nerves tense, and I am "taking down" my prey with my teeth. Holding it in my vise-like jaw, I then drag it home to my family where my neck muscles fire one last time, slamming it down near the cooking fire. I experience a sense of strength and pride at the conclusion of another successful hunt.

This practice appears to be very physical, and the 'energetics' involved may not be initially perceptible. Before you can use your chi with purpose, you must first be able to feel it. When the mind and body are joined in a task, the feelings involved become imprinted onto the mind. Frequent repetition of the physical act will lead to very tangible mental sensations. After putting in some time with hard physical body motion, it becomes easy to see how soft mental imagination and visualization includes the solid, physical "chi feeling." Ultimately, using the mind alone, with no physical movement, will result in "feeling" the chi. Remember, it is best to practice alone in a quiet setting in order to focus on the imagination. Once the feeling becomes natural and spontaneous, add it into your game.

The simplest way to learn energy work is by one-on-one training with a teacher. Learning such techniques from a book alone is possible, but working with an experienced teacher makes for a more rapid and well-rounded learning experience. Experiencing chi transmission and reception is easier when an actual teacher is present—and the student is ready. For beginners attempting to get a feel for chi, I recommend the following schools/systems:

Taichi Tao Center www.taichitaocenter.com

Intended Evolution Fitness 150 www.ifit150.com

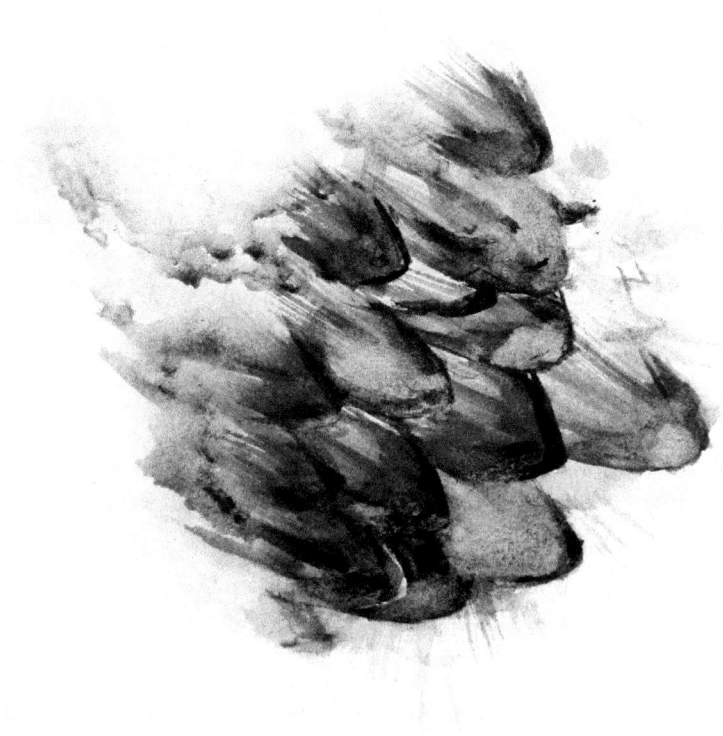

CHAPTER 21
RELAXATION WITH DETERMINATION

If you are serious about your martial arts, consider focusing some of your energy on the teeth and tongue. When teeth and tongue are incorporated into training, the wisdom behind the lips of The Laughing Buddha will become apparent. But The Laughing Buddha does not share his secrets with any who fail to follow these five rules:

Relax Completely
Maintain Teeth Touching Lightly/Teeth Apart
Touch Tip of Tongue to Palate
Observe Posture
Breathe with Diaphragm

1. Relax Completely

How can one relax completely unless one also understands what it is to be completely tense? This is the way of energy—tense, relax, tense, relax, tense, relax. Chronic tension results in pain, disease, and death, but excessive relaxation leads to lethargy, depression, disease, and death. The secret to health, strength, vitality, and longevity is to lead a life of balance within varying degrees of tension and relaxation. During Teeth in Mortal Combat training, one utilizes tension and relaxation of the entire body, with special focus on the head and neck. Use the Predator-X jaw and Hex-Diamond White teeth to take down the prey, pick it up, and drop it at the cook's fire—and then relax. Attack and release. Tense and relax.

The first rule, to relax completely, may seem simple but there are many ways to relax, some more appropriate than others. It might be more accurate to use the term "relax correctly" rather than "relax completely." Learning to relax correctly can require much experimentation by the student and personal attention by an instructor. And one essential prerequisite of learning this skill is putting in a hard day's work.

For years I avoided stressful mental activities, strenuous exercise, and hard physical labor in order to grant myself as much time as possible to attempt to "relax completely." This was certainly another "mistake of inches" that led to my ending miles off course. What I have discovered, as the culmination of twenty-five years of trying to learn how to relax, is that the easiest and quickest way is to first work hard from dawn 'til dusk. At the end of the workday, when you are home and beginning to unwind, spend some time practicing and examining relaxation techniques. This will allow you to have a better understanding of what if feels like to relax and, more importantly, what it *means* to relax. Once you become accomplished at this, and add meditation to the mix, you can then apply the lessons learned into your hard working day—and I mean HARD work! Do not make the mistake of thinking that it is not possible to simultaneously work hard and relax. Work your fingers to the bone. Accomplish something with your life and be of service to the world.

I believe hard work in service will open your heart to the gift of deep relaxation. Remember, your work can become your meditation. Relaxation is a positive side effect of doing work and meditation correctly.

2. Teeth Apart

My tai chi teacher used to say, "The teeth should be lightly touching *and* not touching." Sometimes there was a slight variation: "The teeth should lightly touch *without* touching." I had no idea what he meant and I was paying him well to share his secrets with me. I did notice that he used the word "lightly" in both instructions. There must be some importance to touching *LIGHTLY*. To this day I do not know exactly what he meant. (If anyone can shed light on this for me, I would appreciate an email …)

I can, however, tell you what happens scientifically when one either clenches hard or "lightly" taps the teeth. Scientifically, we know that conscious *light* "tapping" of the teeth is a positive and healthy exercise that stimulates blood circulation in the root and surrounding bone. This helps eliminate the build up of toxins and improves the transport of nutrients to the teeth. Over time, lightly tapping the teeth during conscious exercise leads to greater bone mass and mineral density. Toxins are eliminated, nutrition improved, and overall regeneration and preservation of tissue is enhanced to extend the lifespan of the teeth.

Subconscious *hard* "clenching" over a long period of time leads to an opposite unhealthy result and can contribute to a shortened lifespan for the teeth. Clenching during martial arts training, if not done with caution and understanding, can become a serious tooth and health issue. The Temporal Mandibular Joint (TMJ) is a sensitive area consisting of nerves, arteries, and veins. When the masseter muscle clenches, the mandibular condyle compresses the TMJ joint bi-laminar area against the temporal fossa. Tetanic, tonic, or continuous muscle contraction with spasm of the masseter muscle eventually leads to an outstripping of the blood supply, lactic acid build-up, and fatigue of the muscles that close the jaw. Chronic and subconscious clenching may also harm the vital tissues in the TMJ joint as well as lead to soreness in the masseter and temporalis muscle. Clenching, without appropriate rest and recovery, may lead to pain and inflammation in the masseter and TMJ, and adjoining head, neck, and facial areas. Subconscious chronic clenching, or bruxism, often results in chronic headaches, visual disturbances, ear ringing, arthritis, limited jaw mobility, and loss of teeth.

Bruxism is the leading cause of occlusal trauma. It can result in abnormal tooth occlusal surface wear patterns, abfractions, and is extremely taxing on the tooth surface usually resulting in micro-fractures of the enamel surface. Over time the accumulation of micro-fractures may weaken the tooth enamel to the point of causing major cracks and chips. Often times in the mature adult, there is a non-restorable partial or complete splitting of the root structure resulting in loss of the tooth. This serious consequence is more common if the tooth has been hollowed out by previous decay or dental drilling. Chronic bruxism—clenching and grinding of teeth—is a significant factor in bone resorption, gum recession, and tooth loss.

Misaligned teeth interfere with the natural muscular movements of teeth sharpening. The long term effects could lead to teeth, jaw, head, neck, and shoulder pain. Ask your dentist to evaluate the smoothness of your bite and if there are any occlusive interferences. Consider any occlussal corrections your dentist might suggest, including orthodontics.

The stress of career, work, and relationships are contributing factors to subconscious Bruxism. It is always best to address the problem of Bruxism before painful symptoms surface. Neutralize mental stress and bring balance into your life. Understand the Thegotic Theory of psychosocial suppression and find help in resolving the repression of the natural instinct to sharpen teeth.

Healthy muscles and bones in the jaw are essential. Mandibular Alveolar Bone Mass (MABM) measures interdental bone thickness. Skeletal Bone Mineral Density (BMD) refers to the amount of minerals in the bone such as calcium, magnesium, fluoride, and phosphorous. Greater bone mass and density makes for bone that is stronger and more resistant to fracture. The greater the MABM and BMD, the stronger and more resistant the bone is to stress fracture. Those among us who are desirous of a Predator-X steel jaw should attempt to increase both MABM and BMD with appropriate exercise and nutrition.

And studies have shown that masseter thickness and the number of occluding mandibular teeth were significant determinants of BMD. Masseter thickness occurs when the muscle is exercised and is a natural byproduct of eating hard and chewy foods, but it can also be due to the destructive subconscious habit of grinding and clenching. People with masseter thickness to the extent that it gives the appearance of a "square jaw" might want to examine if it is caused by pathological chronic bruxism or due to eating healthy, hard foods. Martial artists require a strong masseter with thick MABM and hard BMD in order to prevent jaw fracture during combat. Masseter thickness, MABM, and BMD may be increased by either safe teeth tapping or dangerous bruxing.

One way to positively affect the muscles, ligaments, and lymph around the face, jaw, and teeth is "tongue rolling." Tongue rolling stimulates salivary function, which is important for the exchange of minerals and waste between the enamel, dentin, and pulp tissue. It also energetically moves the chi within and around the teeth to increase vital function. This is a common chi kung technique, known to all knowledgeable instructors.

An important component of teeth, and one that is essential to dental health, is enamel. Human enamel is brittle: like glass, it cracks easily, but unlike glass, enamel is able to contain cracks and remain intact for the course of a lifetime. The major reason why teeth do not fracture and break apart is due to the presence of 'tufts'—small, crack-like defects found deep in the tooth at the dentin-enamel junction. These tufted cracks prevent major tooth chips and fractures due to trauma and biting by evenly distributing and absorbing the traumatic force.

Enamel also has a "basket weave" micro structure which protects against crack growth. Teeth possess a self-healing process wherein organic material fills cracks extending from the tufts. This type of infilling bonds opposing crack walls and increases the amount of force needed to break the tooth. Safe teeth tapping utilizes this unique self-healing aspect to rebuild and strengthen teeth. Martial artists make use of this natural crack-healing ability to rebuild and strengthen the body so that they can break baseball bats with their shinbones, or bricks with their hands and heads. Similar results may be obtained through teeth tapping, and a healthy tooth should easily crack walnuts and other hard-shelled foods. If you want to change your glass jaw into one of steel, it helps to understand these modern scientific principles while you incorporate ancient chi kung training techniques. Strong healthy teeth are your main source of resistance training for increasing masseter strength, bone mass, and bone density.

Tapping the teeth and conscious clenching, when practiced correctly, are the beginning techniques of Teeth in Mortal Combat training. Teeth tapping vibrates the hard yet supple tooth structure and associated fluids setting up shock waves that help push the toxic waste out. Teeth tapping also strengthens the tooth structure against the impact of daily biting, chewing, and grinding. Conscious light "tapping" of your teeth improves chi energy and blood circulation through the roots, gums, and bone. Over time, lightly tapping the teeth during exercise leads to greater bone mass and mineral density. Toxins are eliminated, nutrition improved, and overall regeneration and preservation of body tissue is enhanced to extend the lifespan of the teeth. As one progresses, the intensity of tapping and clenching naturally builds, so in order to safely increase masseter thickness and strength, as well as MABM and BMD, healthy molar and premolar teeth are of vital importance.

You may be wondering why most of this section has been devoted to teeth touching even though its title is "Teeth Apart." There is a good reason for this seeming anomaly: I want to emphasize the physical dangers of both conscious and subconscious teeth touching when practiced without guidance. Many people make the mistake of initially biting or tapping with too much force, or acquiring the bad habit of bruxism. Teeth touching is serious business and mistakes can result in permanent damage to your teeth, bone, and jaw.

Training *teeth apart,* however, is very safe and innocuous. The easiest way to train "teeth apart" is to take a few seconds and step away from what you are doing and then "yawn, smile, swallow your saliva, relax." If your mouth is dry, take a sip of water or put something sweet or sour into your mouth. One goji berry or a small piece of lemon peel is all it takes to activate the salivary glands.

There are times throughout the day when your teeth naturally touch or do not touch. For example, when you swallow it is normal for the teeth to lightly touch, but when you yawn, the teeth do not touch. Relax and know that most of the day you are in the groove. See this natural reflex every time you drink a beverage or swallow your saliva. This is the physical level to explain the instruction, "the teeth should be lightly touching and not touching."

If you find it difficult to relax and keep your teeth apart, then focus more on the tongue. Concentrating on the tongue can signal the salivary glands to secrete more saliva—a Yin process—which may then be swallowed so its healing chi may be absorbed by lower dan-tien, signalling the nervous system to restore peace and calm. Pent up repressive emotions melt and the teeth and jaws relax. As a result, the teeth will tend to stay apart, coming together with only the minimum necessary force indicated for proper function ... Life is beautiful!

Masters give such instruction as focusing on the tongue to help the student free the mind from the world of attached thoughts. This is called "taming the wild horse." Placing the focus of the mind on an immediate puzzle does not allow for thoughts of the past or future. It anchors one in the present moment, where the only reality exists.

Conscious awareness of "teeth apart" is necessary for the brain to make the appropriate changes, and in order to be aware of "teeth apart," it helps to first have them touch lightly. Joining a meditation class can be very helpful. You know the old saying, "Success comes with numbers."

Remember the mantra:

Lips Together, Teeth Apart
Relax, Smile and Open Your Heart!

3. Tongue on Palate

Most meditations require lightly placing the tip of the tongue on the upper palate. There are a number of reasons for this: the tongue is a very energy-sensitive muscle and serves as a conduit for language, cognitive thought, and emotional experiences such as suckling, tasting, and sexual pleasure. Activate the mind and the tongue prepares itself to express the thoughts. As previously mentioned, the tongue, heart, and mind are energetically associated, and the tongue also is used to form a bridge connecting the Conception and Governing vessels. But unless the tongue has a purpose during active meditation, it can prove to be a distraction. Assigning this simple task to the tongue allows the mind to remain more focused and makes it easier to find the quiet space within.

A more medical reason to press the tongue on the roof of the mouth is related to sinus problems. It is commonly believed that pressing hard on the upper palate with the thumb of one hand, and then using the palm of the other hand to press firmly on the spot between the eyes, can 'rock' the sinus. Alternating the pressure between the two spots for twenty seconds creates a rocking vibration that will cause some movement of the nasal and vomer (a facial bone just atop the palate) bones to open the sinus and allow congestion to drain. I believe that just pressing the tongue against the roof of the mouth will create a similar effect, allowing the air and energy to circulate more freely through the nose and sinus. A free flow of breath and energy are helpful during both quiet meditation and physical exercise.

The upper palate is a fairly large space and there are various locations, depending on one's purpose, where the tongue tip may be placed. A good starting point is the "cluck" position: make a "clucking" sound and see where the tongue touches the palate in order to produce that sound. (For dental professionals reading this, if the "cluck" feels too "ducky," then perform a zygomatic smile, slide into centric relation, lightly touch the teeth together, and bring the tip of the tongue up to touch the palate somewhere between the central and posterior region. You will have no trouble finding the "sweet" spot as it feels like sipping sweet nectar.) When the tongue is pressed against the roof of the mouth or above the front teeth of the upper palate, the chi is activated and a strong connection between the mind and tongue is established. By holding the tongue in a stable position against the palate, the activated chi can be harnessed and directed for purposes other than speaking.

When the tongue is relaxed and allowed to rest in the center of the mouth without touching the palate, the chi is also activated, but with a different purpose. Thoughts immediately slow down while potential energy accumulates in various storage chambers. This is the difference between active and passive meditation. In both cases, either with the tongue relaxed and not touching the palate, or with the tongue touching the palate, the activity of the mind calms down. In active meditation the quieted mind is prepped, much like drawing an arrow back in a bow, harnessing the energy in preparation to shoot. In passive meditation, the still mind watches the universe move within and without; there is no intention to shoot, but the potential exists and it can change at any moment.

Try it. Close your eyes and relax your tongue and you will notice how quickly your mind softens and relaxes and the chi accumulates. This helps you in your passive meditation. If you are practicing specific active meditations, press the tongue on the roof of the mouth and sense how your energy activates and strengthens. When your tongue touches the upper palate, the elixirs in saliva flow and, when swallowed, drain into and fill lower dan-tien. Use the mind to stoke the fire in the dan-tien in order to purify and transmute the elixir.

The tongue position is reflexively controlled by jaw position (the jaw-tongue reflex). During combat, one needs to protect the jaw by retruding it, or moving and holding it in the most rearward position. This is possible because of the multi-dimensional nature of the TMJ which functions to hold and move the jaw into its many versatile positions. When the mandible is retruded, the tongue reflexively moves into the best position for bridging the upward and downward flowing energy pathways within the oral cavity. In dentistry, this retruded position is called "centric relation."

Swallowing also reflexively moves the tongue into the ideal place for meditation. Many meditations call for one to 'swallow'

192 Teeth In Mortal Combat

imaginary objects such as the sun, moon, flames, watery elixirs, pearls, etc. Swallowing helps one to become more familiar with the tongue's energy and how it engages with the other energies flowing in and around the oral cavity. It is valuable to watch and feel how the different parts of the oral cavity interact while these meditations are performed.

There are many different optimal positions for the tongue to occupy depending on the specific practice. But when involved in mortal combat, the last thing a combatant needs to worry about is tongue placement. One's instinct should take care of this detail, allowing one to focus entirely on survival and victory. During combat, the tongue should instinctively and subconsciously be controlled so as to prevent accidental self-biting. A blow to the face can force the mandible upward with great momentum, causing a severe bite to the tongue. Placing the tongue upward against the center of the palate, or curling it down behind the lower front teeth, will prevent such a traumatic injury. This is another reason to practice pressing it against the roof of the mouth. If this instinct is repressed, repetitious practice is necessary to reawaken this technique.

When preparing for combat, it is important to marshal all of the various instinctive survival energies. Like a complex energy grid at times of intense overload, certain energy pathways are required to shut down in order to direct the maximum amount of energy to the meridians and organs used for self-preservation; having active digestive energy during a fight for life is counter-productive. (During training it is necessary to be conscious of the amount of chi and pressure in the various meridians in order to prevent damage—in the form of an 'energetic aneurysm'—from occurring. Working one-on-one with a qualified instructor is vital to adequately mastering this aspect of chi management.)

When training for mortal combat, the tendency is to bite and clench the teeth to extremes, which can lead to damaging the teeth. One method to solve this problem is to rely on the Yin energy of the tongue to contain the exuberant Yang energy of the teeth. During peak periods of physical practice, press the tongue hard against the roof of the mouth. When the tongue is pressed into the upper palate with sufficient strength, the teeth are unable to clench with maximum force. The pressure with the tongue will vary depending on the practice, and with trial and error it is possible to achieve the proper and comfortable balance between tongue pressure and teeth biting force. Another trick to keep the teeth from clenching too hard is to bring the teeth lightly together and then inhale through the mouth and front teeth as if sucking the air into the mouth through the spaces between the teeth. It should create a "hissing" sound when the tongue is properly placed.

The only appropriate time to have the teeth biting down with maximum force is when there is something between the jaws, such as a hunted animal, or an opponent's body part. During training, when there is nothing between the teeth and tooth-to-tooth contact is being made, make certain to press the tongue against the palate with enough pressure to prevent compressive bite force injury to the teeth. *Never, for any reason or at any time, clench to the limit during visualization and imagination exercises.* This could easily cause dental-facial trauma such as cracked teeth, broken fillings and crowns, TMJ injury, and lockjaw.

I believe that even though the tongue channels energy more efficiently while in contact with the roof of the mouth, there may be more distraction in telling a novice to do so than there is benefit to be gained. At the very beginning of your practice, it is acceptable to just let the tongue relax and have it rest behind the top two front teeth. As you proceed, integrate the more complicated techniques in a logical, comfortable progression in order to avoid injury.

4. Posture

Development of one's posture depends upon genetics, the birth experience as one enters the world, and the effects of emotions on the body as we grow and mature. Many books addressing perfect posture have been written, but reading is not enough: one must first be aware of posture and then consciously work to correct it. My personal experiences with working on posture may be of some help.

I tried for twenty-five years to consciously improve my posture by tucking in the tailbone, pulling up the perineum, imagining a string attached to and pulling up the crown point at the top of my skull, balancing books on the top of the head, etc. These methods were effective—up to a point—but nothing worked as well as simple sprinting and walking on my toes. I became more aware of my posture after walking on the balls and toes of my feet for two or three miles at a time. My awareness improved further by sprinting short distances of about fifty yards on the balls of my feet. I did both of the above at least twice a week for several months. Try it and observe your results.

It is interesting to note that babies innately know to begin ambulation with the "toddler walk" and to run on the balls of their feet. As they mature, they start to imitate their parents and begin walking heel-to-toe. Which is correct or preferable: heel-to-toe or toe-to-heel? I am not qualified to answer that question, but I do believe there is benefit in watching babies use what the gurus call "no mind." I vary my walking style in order to hone my awareness.

Try walking and sprinting on the balls of your feet. It works wonders to improve posture!

5. Breathe with Diaphragm

Full breathing with the diaphragm is the fundamentally most important exercise for one to perform in order to achieve progress in all areas of chi development. Many various types of breathing exercises that have originated in China and India are now being taught and practiced in the West. In order to gain valuable exposure to as many of these as possible, it is necessary to work with a teacher who has a strong background in chi kung and/or pranayama breathing techniques. At the time of this writing, David Blaine holds the world record for holding his breath and a number of his excellent breathing exercises may be found online.

I strongly suggest that you find a teacher who will safely guide you through the finer points of breathing exercises. One bit of advice I can contribute is to place your hand on your stomach and feel the abdomen expand outward with the inhale and contract inward with the exhale. In some practices, the desired effect is the opposite—the stomach expands outward on the exhale and contracts inward with the inhale.

I would like to share with you an exercise that will enhance your awareness of breath and chi and simultaneously benefit the diaphragm, teeth and nervous system:

1. Purchase a pair of Vibram Five Finger, FeelMax Niesa, mocassin, or any other similar style of barefoot running or walking shoe. This type of shoe is the best that I have found to help me connect with the energy of the earth while still protecting the soles of my feet.

2. Stand comfortably and clasp the fingers of your hands together and rest them on top of the head.

3. Keep the teeth apart and lightly press the tip of the tongue onto the roof of the mouth.

4. Breathe through the nose. If you are unable to breathe
    smoothly through the nose, breathe through the mouth.
5. Tense the perineum slightly—and definitely avoid clenching
    tightly—so you can locate it and feel the energy move up the
    spine.
6. Relax the entire body—and pay special attention to relax-
    ing the abdomen—bend the knees slightly, and start walking
    very slowly backwards.
7. Coordinate your breaths with each step. Inhale while taking
    one step backward, exhale on the next step backward. Repeat
    in a rhythmic pattern. (As you become comfortable with this
    technique, you can play with different rhythms of breathing
    and stepping.)
8. Continue in this manner until you have your balance and are
    relatively relaxed.
9. Relax the abdomen, allow the teeth to touch lightly, and step
    backward slowly. With each step, inhale the breath in stages,
    a little at a time: breathe first into the perineum, then the
    lower abdomen, and continue to inhale in increments until
    the breath fills the upper abdomen, the solar plexus, middle
    chest area, and continue this process until the upper chest
    and shoulders are completely filled with air. At this point the
    entire torso, from perineum to shoulders, is completely filled
    with air.
10. With the next step *explode* all of the air out through the nose
    or mouth in this manner: pull up on the perineum, con-
    tract the abdomen inward toward the spine, compress the
    rib cage, pull the shoulders down, and interlock the fingers
    strongly down onto the head. Most importantly, the abdo-
    men should fire backwards like a piston, striking against the
    front of the spine.

11. Repeat this pattern until you tire of it and then turn around, relax, and start walking forward. Continue breathing and exploding in a more relaxed manner and with a reduced measure of horsepower. Imagine that when you begin the exercise you are in neutral, release the clutch and explode into first gear, then second, third, and fourth gear. When you tire, turn around and start walking forward and shift into fifth gear, coasting comfortably while you regain your composure and energy. The piston does not have to slap the spine while you are in fifth gear. When you feel re-energized, turn around and start walking backward again and repeat the steps.

12. You should spend most of your time enjoying the recovery stage in fifth gear, coasting comfortably while taking in the fresh air and enjoying nature. When you feel the time is right for another explosion, turn around and begin walking backward, drop down into neutral and explode with all of your accessible horsepower into first gear, second, and so on until turning around and walking forward again in 5th gear.

Fifth gear is most enjoyable and it is very important that you spend most of your time there. Figure 5–10% of the time for first gear, 10–20% for second, third, and fourth combined, and 70–80% for fifth gear. Use this opportunity to become more in touch with your chi: when you tire, do not use your will power and force yourself to drop down and explode again into first gear. Wait until your chi "tells" you that recovery is complete, the tank is topped off, and the engine and driver are ready. Recognize and pay attention to your chi communicating with you. The mind and will are very powerful and may easily convince you to start too soon, before the chi is ready. *Listen to your chi in order to gain the most benefit.*

Forward walking is where the barefoot running shoe reveals its significant advantage over conventional walking, jogging, or running shoes. As you step forward, hit the heel HARD on the ground. The impact will transfer earth energy through the thin rubber sole and send a vibration upward through the skeletal bones from the heel to the leg, up through the spine to the neck and skull, finally connecting with the mandible by way of the TMJ. The vibration ends with the teeth gently clashing against each other and the teeth will begin to vibrate in rhythm with the steps. This creates a cool experience that is very healthy and invigorating for the whole body, including the brain.

You will discover remarkable benefits for the teeth. When you feel the teeth vibrating, know that your brain cells are also are being affected in a positive way by the vibrational frequency. Your entire central nervous system begins to rewire itself into a higher level of potential energy conduction.

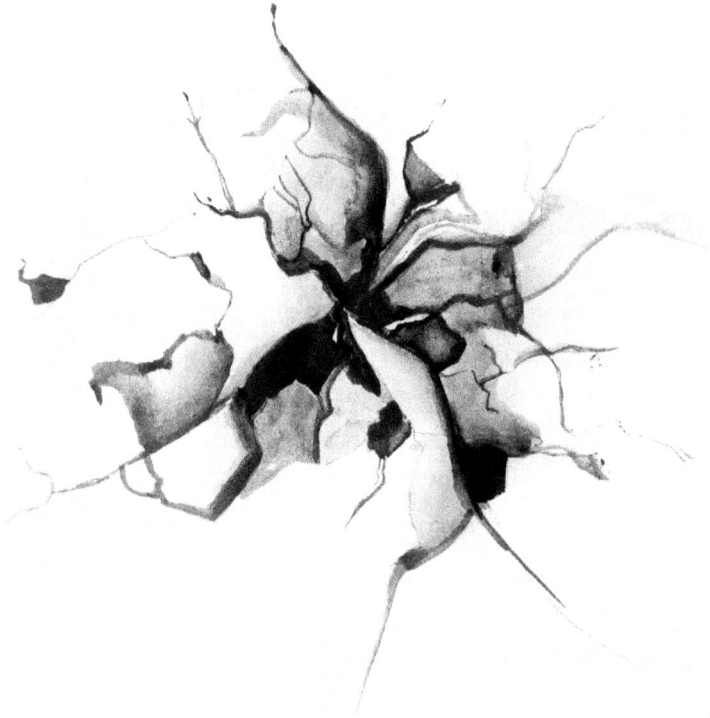

Chapter 22
ATHLETIC MOUTH GUARDS AND HELMETS

The conventional wisdom has it that athletic mouth guards are important for safety and protection of the mouth and teeth, and that mouth guards are an essential piece of protective gear for athletes who play contact sports. Accordingly, an athletic mouth guard not only protects the teeth, but the soft tissue around the mouth area that may be damaged by the teeth. I agree, in a limited way, with these statements.

Helmets are likewise viewed as essential prophylaxis for preventing head injuries. An estimated 1.6 to 3.8 million recreation-related concussions are sustained annually in the United States, many of them on football fields. When children and teens suffer a concussion, they must be strictly monitored and their activities restricted. They should never under any circumstances return to the field of play, and no cognitive activities such as reading and studying for school, text messaging, video games or television are allowed until they have fully recovered.

The problem today is that sports-related concussions in children and athletes often go unrecognized and often do not receive proper respect for their potential seriousness. A concussion is actually—mild traumatic brain injury. A recent study found that if a child is given a diagnosis of concussion, parents treat it more lightly than if it is spoken more correctly as "mild traumatic brain injury." The change in language by medical doctors could help protect the child from returning to school sooner than recommended. One study of U.S. college athletes who had concussions indicated suppressed brain function more than three years later.

Newly redesigned helmets show promise to further protect the skull from splitting, although they still cannot prevent an athlete's brain from rattling around inside the skull like a scrambled yolk inside an eggshell. But more and more studies are revealing that mouth guards, helmets, etc. are NOT protecting contact sport athletes from long-term negative health consequences. *They are only providing a false sense of security.*

American football is one of the most dangerous sports on the planet because of the false sense of safety that mouth guards and helmets generate. Repetitive hits to the body, even with protective body armor, usually impart a concussive force to the skeletal structure, spinal cord, and brain. An athlete, after just one season, can end up with permanent physical and mental damage that will go unnoticed until later in life. It is little wonder that professional football players have recently begun to donate their brains to science so that the long-term effects of multiple concussions may be studied.

Australian Rules Football has a no-helmet rule, yet their players have twenty-five percent fewer head injuries than helmeted American players. This one statistic alone should raise a red flag about the consequences of wearing a helmet. The false sense of security a helmet provides drives athletes to 'spear' opponents with their heads. Spearing is very dangerous to all involved, and head injuries, immediate and delayed, almost always result. In my opinion, helmets should be banned from American football. And until that comes to pass, spearing with the helmet should be disciplined by banning the offending player from the sport for life.

Head injuries are also much more likely to occur when a fatigued or injured player enters the game, and in the world of multi-million dollar pro contracts, little is done to prevent this from happening. Head injuries, even if asymptomatic at game time, may remain passive in nature until they erupt like a boil years later. Symptoms of brain concussion injuries, often dormant when young, begin to show themselves in many athletes by the time they reach their early thirties.

If athletes must wear mouth guards to protect their teeth, then they are playing with fear, fatigue, or injury. If one is fearless and fresh, one's reflexes will be fully active and one's chi should protect against serious injuries. A player with fresh, active chi does not need a mouth guard or a helmet. I believe there would be fewer head and teeth injuries if players were trained to use their chi to protect themselves from injury. Of course, this scenario is dependent upon the assumption that athletes are aware of their chi and paying attention to its subtle messages as to whether it is fatigued or unable to fully protect them. Coaches are certainly also responsible for keeping fatigued and injured players out of the game. Common sense combined with heightened chi awareness is the solution to many serious athletic injuries.

In my opinion, American football—as it is played with helmet, body padding, and mouth guard—comes very close to fitting the description of mortal combat because of the possible long-term negative effects on the brain. **I support mortal combat in only two instances: one is in life and death situations, and the other is in training for survival.** *Teeth in Mortal Combat* prepares a warrior for those specific scenarios; it is not to be used for sport and play. I do not believe in or support spectator sports involving anything close to mortal combat for amusement. Survival for one's life is VERY serious business, not entertainment to be had with beer and chips on the side.

Returning to the topic of mouth guards, I would like to highlight some facts about their usage and how they ultimately interfere with the development of chi in the teeth, jaws, and tongue. The TMJ is the most active joint in the body, as it is used for breathing, chewing, swallowing, and speaking. Keeping the joint healthy and free of injury should be of primary importance to martial artists, but wearing a mouth guard does not help in this regard. On the contrary, it actually interferes with the body's natural innate patterns of self-preservation.

First, it is important to note that when we bite down, we are not literally biting *down*. The top teeth do not bite downward, rather it is the bottom teeth and jaw that are biting upward. Upward biting plays an important role in the development and utilization of chi in the mouth because it requires one to draw upon the upward flowing energy of the conception vessel. The downward flowing energy of the governing vessel stabilizes the head and keeps the upper teeth positioned for contact with the lower. When the two energies meet, there is a dynamic whirlpool of potential energy in the head, neck, and mouth area.

(So how did the phrase "bite down" originate? We do know that the idiom "bite the dust" means to fall down dead. My guess is that many thousands of years ago, long before the advent of bows or firearms, combatants who bit the dust did so because their opponent forcefully smashed them down to the ground, similar to the meaning of the phrase "take down" used in wrestling. The phrase "bite down" was eventually modernized and applied to any biting of the jaw and teeth.)

I believe there is the memory of our original ancient ancestor stored in the energetic blueprint of our jaw, and that we can tap into it during mortal combat. And I am quite certain that this ancestor possessed a biting mechanism that was ripe with chi potential and likewise depended on the jaw and teeth for self-defense during mortal combat to a tremendous extent. In order to awaken this powerful function within ourselves, we can do some simple exercises and visualizations. The tongue, as mother to the teeth, plays a role in this awakening process by helping to open up the entire system, including the psyche, to respond to commands. It releases inner strength and abolishes fear.

When one wears a mouth guard, the teeth and lower jaw are splinted into a fixed position and the tongue is prevented from freely touching the teeth. One of the first rules in chi development is to allow the mind, body, and spirit to relax, be flexible, and move freely.

(Naturally, if one is injured or disabled and needs to wear some type of a cast, splint, or brace in order to heal an injury, there are methods available to access healing chi while one is bound by these medical necessities. An injured player, however, should never be allowed onto the playing field as this only puts the weakened player in harm's way and interferes with the healing process. A healthy, fully capable athlete should, on the other hand, never wear a cast, brace, or padding into the arena. If the brace or padding is being worn to avoid possible injury, then it might be time to examine the purpose of the game. Is the game designed to uplift the human spirit and condition? In what ways do the rules advance or hinder the emotional and spiritual growth of the player? What is the relationship between player and spectator? Does the spectator gain twisted pleasure in seeing pain and bloodshed on the field of play?)

One of the beautiful qualities of the tongue is that it communicates with the energy system of the entire body through its contact with the teeth, which have meridians of every organ system in the body running through them. Rubbing the tip of the tongue against all of the tooth surfaces is not only a way to clean the teeth, but it is the method through which the mother tongue connects with the whole body. Rubbing the teeth is also pleasurable to the tongue and strengthens and stimulates it. The salivary glands begin to secrete a higher volume of elixir into the mouth, lubricating the tongue and teeth for even greater pleasure. If you desire a happy, healthy tongue, stimulate it daily by rubbing it against your teeth. Mouth guards serve only to interfere with this natural pleasure.

The universal rule is that a chain is only as strong as its weakest link. This is why we must pay special attention to the jaw if our goal is to increase physical strength. For overall maximum physical output, every part of the body has to function at its optimum ability. In order to kick, punch, or block to maximum effect, the jaw must be freely held in its ideal functioning position so that no link is kinked. The chi must be unrestricted and flowing with full potential through every link in the chain. And in order for the chi to fully protect the teeth and jaw, the mandible must also be perfectly positioned. This position varies according to the posture of the whole body, whether leaning forward, backward, to the left, to the right, stooping, crouching or standing on one leg. The lower jaw position of greatest strength will vary, depending on the angle of the head on the cervical spine. Mouth guards in this situation will interfere with freedom of movement.

The strength of the masseter muscle is directly related to the position of the mandible within the space of the TMJ, and protrusive force directions gain the highest relative activation of the masseter. The posterior deep muscle region of the masseter seems to possess the most active fibers during clenching and biting. This means that one must move the lower jaw slightly forward to find the location of greatest available strength, or 'sweet spot', for the task at hand.

And essential to correct positioning of the jaw, the TMJ is one of the most complex joints in the body. All body parts move with some rotation and circular motion and the jaw is no different; it opens and closes with more than a simple hinged motion. When the jaw is searching for the sweet spot, it will maneuver on multiple axes in a manner that cannot be seen by the naked eye. When the teeth and mandible are locked into a mouth guard, there is no opportunity for the jaw to search for and vibrate into the sweet spot. Finding the sweet spot for maximum strength happens subconsciously, instinctively, reactively, and instantaneously, through constant adjustments to changes in posture and the angle of the head on the cervical spine. The mandible must be free to glide in all directions in order to chomp into the prize with maximum force. It also is a vital link that must remain unimpeded so that other parts of the body can deliver the maximum output of energy—an impossibility if one is saddled with a restrictive mouth guard. Although professional athletes wear mouth guards that are custom made by dentists, it is not possible for the dentist to locate or duplicate the floating sweet spot in an appliance.

Do not rely on helmets, padding, and mouth guards to protect your body, as they only impart a false sense of security at best. They cannot teach your chi to *explode outward*. If you choose to nurture your inner self and strengthen your physical body through athletic endeavors, then participate in sports that give you the freedom to achieve those ends. Find a sport that enables you to access and learn from your chi while simultaneously developing and protecting it. Avoid sports that place your chi in harm's way. Use your chi wisely.

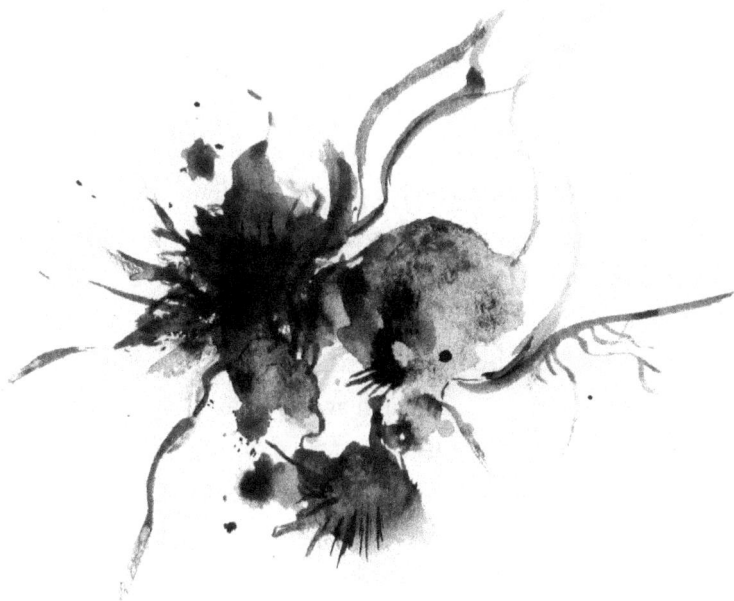

CHAPTER 23
WINE AND DREAMS

Professor Cheng Man-ch'ing was considered, by many, to be the "Mater of Five Excellencies," including Chinese medicine, tai chi chuan, calligraphy, painting, and poetry. In the United States he was most popular for his martial arts ability of unleashing power through his thumbs. When asked how he learned the ability to transfer chi power through an opponent, he would say that *he had a dream in which his arms fell off.* In my humble opinion, dreams are often used to explain away mysterious secrets that a person does not want to share with you. For example, where did I glean the information that has become *Teeth in Mortal Combat?* Well, most of it presented in dreams...

I have listened to a number of eyewitness accounts from American and Chinese martial artists who have studied in China. According to them, many of the chi masters in China drink alcohol as if it were water, smoke tobacco like chimneys, and use narcotics such as opium. This is not surprising considering the fact that, based on evidence uncovered at archaeological sites, opium appears to be a substance of long-standing ritual significance. Anthropologists have speculated that ancient priests may have used the drug as a proof of healing power. Wine, hemp and hallucinogenics are other intoxicants used by spiritual seekers to access higher planes of knowledge. When someone tells me that they acquired information in a dream, I am always interested in learning about the circumstances around the dream-state. I doubt very much that this occurs during the typical REM dream-state experienced by most people every night.

I want to share an epiphany with you, one not associated with a dream-state: when I imagined that my arms had fallen off and I began to visualize fighting a wild animal with my teeth, *a whole new world of possibilities opened up for me.* After I visualized fighting with my teeth and began to incorporate an intense zygomatic smile into my practice, the power of the Laughing Buddha filled my head, neck, oral cavity, teeth, and jaws. My top and bottom halves connected with my bottom, right side separated from left side, front became clear against back.

You, too, can have a similar experience: Visualize your arms shackled behind your back and fight with your teeth. Hiss like the snake, prowl like the tiger, growl with the lion. Use your teeth to take down, choke, pull, push, pin against a tree, throw into the river. Take the yoke between your teeth and pull the plow freely. Work the field. Lift the earth, swing the moon, fish the stars. Release an invisible net of chi from your mouth, hook and sinker baited with instinct.

This is what I call a "Dance with Fierce Hoopla!"

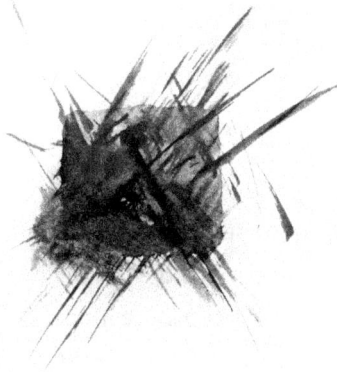

Chapter 24
BASIC TRAINING INSTRUCTION

Training teeth and jaws involves certain risks and I strongly caution everyone interested in attempting to use the exercises portrayed on my website, *www.Tooth-Fight.com,* to first undergo complete and thorough dental and medical examinations. *This chapter contains the only written instructions for the exercise training videos on my website. Watching the videos in combination with reading this chapter should answer all of your questions on how to practice.* **Attempting to study and practice the exercises shown on the videos without reading this book—or vice versa—may be harmful to your health.**

Fresh air is an essential ingredient to a healthy training session. If practicing inside, crack open a window or door. It is preferable to train barefoot or wear an ultra-thin soled shoe like a moccasin or barefoot running shoe. Avoid urinating after training for at least 20 minutes to help prevent dissipating any chi accumulated during the session.

It is recommended to use silk fabric for this training. Silk is a natural protein fiber very similar to human hair and our bodies respond far better to silk than they do to synthetic products. Natural amino acids in the silk fiber are very similar to human hair. It is naturally hypoallergenic and is mold and mildew resistant due to its ability to wick away moisture. Because of its smooth surface, its frictional coefficient is only 7.4%, which is the lowest among all fibers. It is relatively resistant to aging. It is best to buy silk colored with natural dyes and dyestuffs made from plants, minerals, and insects. The silk should be about three feet wide and the length of your body. Fold the silk onto itself three times in order to get a comfortable fit.

Lesson One: Warm-up

1a) Be certain as many teeth as possible are biting into the silk. Hold the silk with your hands below your head. As you inhale slowly, pull the silk upward and extend the neck comfortably as far back as possible. Hesitate a moment, then exhale slowly and completely as you pull the chin down toward your chest. Hesitate a moment then repeat several times.

1b) This time repeat the instructions in 1a) holding the silk in your hands above your head.

2a) Face straight ahead, keep both arms outstretched at your sides, and inhale completely. Exhale slowly as you pull the silk to the right as far as your neck will allow, then try turning a bit more to see behind you as you completely expel all the remaining air in your lungs. Hesitate a moment, then begin inhaling slowly while using your teeth to pull the silk back to the starting position. Hesitate a moment and then repeat again several times.

2b) Follow the same procedure turning the head to the opposite side.

Lesson Two: Squat and Rise

Be absolutely sure that you tie your silk securely to the doorknob and that the door is firmly closed, locked, or bolted and that it is impossible for the door to come open. Clear the area behind you so that if your bite grip, silk tie knot, door lock or jamb accidentally are compromised, there will be no injury should you fall backward.

Begin by standing close to the door and maintaining a fairly vertical body position while holding the silk with both hands. As you become stronger and more confident, increase the backward lean and release your grip on the silk. Eventually and **ideally, you want to keep your hands folded over your lower abdomen.**

Open your eyes wide and maintain a zygomatic smile. Inhale completely and then slowly exhale as you squat down as far as comfort allows. The motion should be teeth pulling the chin towards the chest. Expel all the air from your lungs, hesitate, and then slowly rise as you breathe into and try to expand your lower abdomen. When you approach your starting position, arch your spine and neck backward as the shoulders pull back and complete your inhale by expanding the chest wall in all directions as much as comfort allows. Hesitate a moment, then repeat squatting and rising several times.

Lesson Three: Completion—Sealing Chi

Stand with feet apart slightly wider than shoulder width. Imagine a heavy barbell resting at your feet and that a weighted object such as a heavy pillow is between your teeth. The teeth DO NOT clench! Breathe through your teeth and create a 'shi' sound.

Eyes are wide open with a zygomatic smile and knees are slightly bent. Inhale completely, then exhale and bend over to pick up the heavy barbell while holding the weighted pillow between your teeth. *The teeth ALWAYS lead the movement. In other words, the teeth lift the pillow just slightly before you pick up the barbell. Always keep your focus on the teeth.* Inhale and pull the barbell to your waist and fling the pillow up and behind your head. **Your spine and neck are arched back, shoulders are pulled back, and your chest is full of air.** Hold your breath as long as possible while you swallow any saliva in your mouth down into your lower dan-tien. (If your mouth is dry, try to force a swallow into your dan-tien or lower abdomen. It is normal to adjust your head and neck from the extended position in order to swallow.) While still firmly holding the barbell at your waist, exhale as you bend forward and use your teeth to whip the pillow from behind your head and slam it to the ground. The imaginary barbell always remains in your hands. Exhale completely and repeat the motion up and back, hold your breath, swallow, and slam the pillow down.

At the point where you cannot swallow anymore, continue with a couple more movements without the swallow.

Always end the exercise in the physical stance you started from: standing straight up with knees slightly bent, but with a final seal where you force a complete exhale by pulling the shoulders forward and down while simultaneously pulling up the hui-yin/perineum and contracting the lower abdomen.

AND REMEMBER: THE TEETH ALWAYS lead the movement. (Imagine a large whip stock between your teeth as you control the whip.)

When you tire, take a short break and then repeat a few more times until your chi tells you it is time to end. The best time to end is when you are beginning to feel slightly tired, but still energized, happy, and fulfilled. Focus on any good feelings you experience as you recover. Tell yourself, "Golly, this feels good." Enjoy the moment of increased vital energy.

Chapter 25
LIVE AGAIN—TOTALLY FREE!

The martial arts are intended to be a tough, mean, no holds barred combat for survival. Sharp teeth and massive jaws, when developed for martial arts, are lethal weapons born of pure animal instinct. In my opinion, nothing displays more clearly the most fearsome wildness in man's nature than his usage of jaws and teeth for assault and self-defense.

Spectators at today's sporting events do not even flinch when one athlete combatant breaks an opponent's arm, jaw, wrist, or gouges an eye. However, if one athlete uses teeth to rip into the flesh, muscle or sinew of another, the media and fans are quick to brand the offender as a barbarian or, even worse, something sub-human. One has to ask why society bans the use of teeth in self-defense. The awareness and development of the basic instinct of biting for self-defense is stifled at an early age and propriety insists that the awesome and brutal capabilities of teeth and jaws are not even proper subjects for discussion in 'polite society'. What is behind this subjugation, oppression and control of natural instinct?

The taboo on biting is world-wide, and many colorful theories have been contrived to support the various reasons for universal complicity. The theory that I find most interesting—from a mechanical, physiological, biological, and energetic point of view— is revealed in the musings of Reversing the Curse by Jean-Claude Koven. According to Koven, the Anunnuki were an alien species that visited Earth at the time when our solar system was beginning to form. They needed to mine our gold, ship it back to their mother planet and, through an elaborate process, disperse it into their atmosphere in order to restore habitable oxygen levels. The mine laborers rebelled at some point and the Anunnuki leaders decided to replace them with one of Earth's own native species, homo erectus. This solution proved unsatisfactory so the Anunnuki performed genetic engineering to splice genes from our own homo erectus with their native genes. The result was a hybrid species, homo sapiens, which proved perfect for mining.

But there were further problems with interbreeding and uncontrolled population growth. War broke out and the Anunnuki decided on a plan to tame the uncontrollable new species they created in order to allow peace to prevail. They deliberately engineered a genetic code into homo sapiens that would transform their new pool of mining slaves into a more docile, programmable, and controllable group. This mechanism has remained in the human genetic makeup ever since. The engineered gene causes the cervical Atlas (C-1) to dislocate, creating an energy blockage in the spinal column along with a host of physical and mental disturbances.

According to Koven, to this day ninety-nine percent of earth's population is still subject to this ancient curse. The solution is to have the Atlas adjusted back into its perfect position through physical therapy. Chiropractors, doctors, shamans, and practitioners of Atlas Profilax are specially trained to reverse the curse. Ozone injections near the site may also prove to be beneficial.

I have undergone this procedure and can testify to its remarkable healing effects in relieving twenty-five years of pain and stiffness in my neck. Chi kung had helped to loosen and relieve my pain somewhat, but the Atlas Profilax therapy completely corrected and eliminated the pain for a period of three months. One year later I had the procedure done again with the same results. Although the results did not 'hold' for more than three months, the therapy left me with a loose and pain-free neck for a while. I believe the therapy is effective because it releases muscular and tendinous fascial stress, thereby improving blood and lymph oxygenation and allowing sufficient detox of inflammatory substances and complete oxygenation of the injured site. Unfortunately, there are no practitioners of Atlas Profilax within one thousand miles of my home. I am fairly certain that if I was able to have the procedure repeated on a regular basis, my neck would completely and permanently heal.

A dislocated C-1 (Atlas) can certainly affect the continuous free flow of chi into the head, neck, teeth, and jaws, making the Anunnuki curse a viable theory regarding how man has lost the energetic connection with his teeth. Studies show that a misplaced Atlas can disrupt blood flow to the brain stem, setting up an inflammatory process. A misaligned Atlas can also cause a loss of blood circulation to the brain, blood pressure problems, and hinder cerebrospinal fluid circulation and pressure, but it is known that hypertension may be reversed by correcting an Atlas dislocation. A correctly aligned Atlas may well be the KEY to a full recovery to health. The Anunnuki story offers an interesting theory, but the unanswered question still remains:

"Why did humans lose their energetic connection to their teeth?"

In Oriental medicine the kidneys rule the teeth, bones, marrow, and nerves. The role of the kidneys is to store life essence and maintain strong will power. The ability to use our will power to express our unique creativity is dependent on good kidney energy. Strong Kidney Chi gives us the resolve to overcome fear and to pursue our goals. If the kidney energy is weak, our sense of purpose is shaky and we are easily distracted. If the use of teeth, in any way, is suppressed or repressed, the Kidney Chi will also be suppressed and repressed. Likewise, if the circular flow of kidney energy to and from the tooth is disrupted in any way, the will power will weaken. And when a tooth is extracted, the kidney energy is depleted and needs to be restored.

Freud suggested that tooth-loss dreams were about—*surprise*—castration. Women also have these dreams, so castration may be gender specific. The general theme in tooth-loss dreams may have to do with a sense of safety, or fear of a loss of self-sufficiency. (In conscious reality, losing a tooth by accident or disease may promote future negative fear-based decision. And such decisions are not in one's best interest and are certainly not in keeping with the way of the warrior.) Castration leads to weakened male energy and castrated males become more docile and less aggressive and have a dampened sense of ambition. Every time I extract a tooth in my dental practice, I have the very uncomfortable feeling that I am castrating the patient. Now you understand one of the reasons why we dentists are so dedicated to saving teeth, why we passionately preach the prevention of tooth and gum disease.

An interesting scientific fact is that teeth 'jiggle' up and down in synchrony with the arterial pulse. Vascular blood pressure within the tooth's arterial network propels the tooth into a positive, outward moving thrust with each heartbeat. There is deep symbolism here: one can suggest that the **teeth connect with will power** and help to drive the positive outward energy of the evolving human consciousness forward. If one's awareness is flowing freely without disruption, one then has the ability to realize one's full potential. Blocking the chi from fully connecting with the teeth, or suppressing and repressing the use of teeth in any way, can be a barrier to self-realization.

In line with this theory, disrupting the flow of chi to the teeth and jaw could suppress a person's will power and ability to freely follow their internal dreams. Someone with insufficient tooth chi will have a difficult time defending themselves from aggressive, controlling dictators. It is easy to see why an overbearing ruler, parent, spouse, or friend could either purposefully or unconsciously endorse artificial taboos on the use of teeth. The 'freedom' of others is dangerous in the eyes of a controlling and power-driven individual.

We can now begin connecting the dots based on science:
— *Teeth are Linked with Kidney Chi and Will Power*
— *A Dislocated Cervical C-1/Atlas Constricts Blood Flow to the Brain Stem, Head, and Teeth*
— *Tooth Loss and/or Limited Capacity due to Constricted Chi Flow is a Symbol for Castration*
— *Docile Personality Combined with Lack of Ambition may be the Result of a Suppressed and/or Repressed Instinct for Defensive Biting*

Docility coupled with a lack of ambition and weakened will power all contribute to the creation of a populace that is easily controlled and afraid to defend itself—qualities despots find desirous in their servants. Psychological and behavioral modification using social taboos renders people more docile and malleable. All the more reason for rulers to create, support and enforce dis-empowering taboos. Man has created many socially driven taboos, and the restrictions on the use of teeth in self-defense stifles the awareness and expression of personal freedoms and inherent rights. A society that unquestioningly accepts the myriad social taboos imposed upon it may find itself at the mercy of a supreme authority willing to subjugate all sense of individual self-determination. We may never discover the true origin of taboos on biting.

What is important is awareness of the SOLUTIONS that can free us from the existing universal suppression and repression of this basic instinct.

When we move beyond unproven theories of world domination, we see that teeth hold a sacred responsibility in the evolution of life. Tooth and jaw are certainly critical parts of human anatomy. Tooth, being the hardest substance in the body, is naturally the oldest surviving fossil relic known to man, dating back five hundred million years. I think that there must be a good reason for this amazing resilience. Could it be that nature chose the tooth to hold secrets to man's existence that no other part of the body can preserve? Secrets securely locked and protected by the thick enamel casing of a tooth, secrets about our existence that are yet to be discovered?

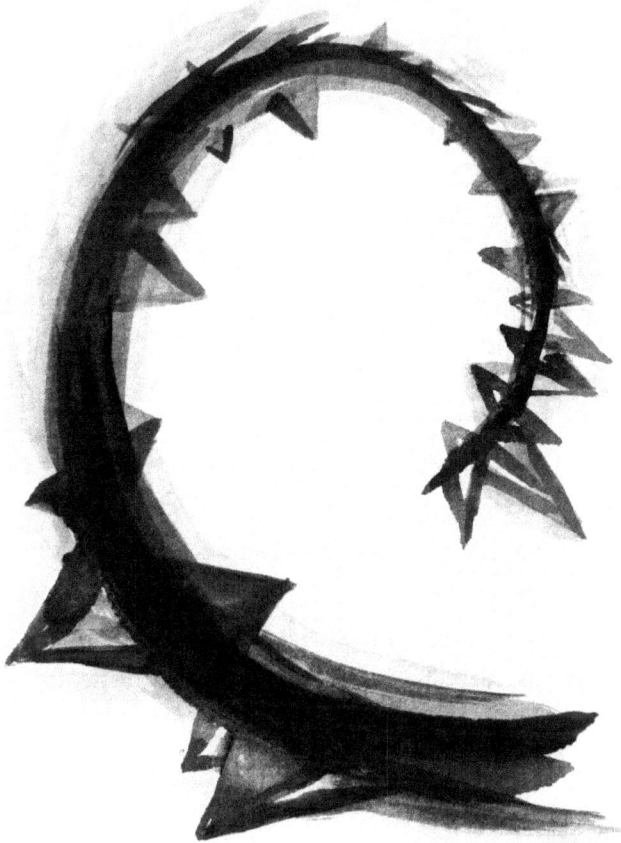

EPILOGUE

During battle to the death in prehistoric days, it is a certainty that these struggles were fought "tooth and nail." Original primal energy was necessarily tapped in order to ensure victory in a vicious fight for life. When a victim is losing the struggle and near death, the last bit of strength remaining will usually go to a futile bite to any exposed and accessible flesh. The mouth is the receptacle for vast amounts of this original primal energy and it is this chi that remains the focus in this book. The sacred mouth sips sweet honey nectar chi, but it can also spit out lethal venomous energy and with its beautiful tongue and teeth can viciously swallow up the life force of another, turning them into slaves, ending their days here on earth.

Man depends on the mouth, teeth, and jaws to feed himself. Early man likely chewed small game such as turtle, frog, snake, fish, bird, and mouse. He did not have the means, at that time, to successfully bring down large game. He certainly could not inflict a lethal bite into the neck of an antelope, wild cat, deer, hog, or other large game animal. Yet his mouth was vital to survival and was packed with large reservoirs of chi, more so than today. That is why I recommend the practice of enhancing the chi of the teeth, tongue, and jaw. One unlocks GREAT potential to increase vital energy and fighting skills by returning to the source.

The first breath of life enters the mouth; mother's milk is taken in at the mouth; the first meal is prepared by chewing with the mouth; the first meaningful sexual encounter usually begins with the mouth. It is the beautiful energy of the mouth that accelerates the breath of life into our dreams and the life and dreams of our brothers and sisters. And so neglect and misuse of the mouth necessarily engenders weakness and disease.

There is a spiritual power to the teeth, tongue, and jaw that is both respected and feared by those who know it. Many cultures from the past held deer teeth in high regard and buried their dead with them, and to date archaeologists have uncovered graves fifteen thousand years old containing hundreds of red deer canine teeth. Deer teeth are spiritual relics that symbolized hunting and one's ability to provide for others. It makes good sense, in today's world, to focus and meditate on our own teeth in the hope that we may perhaps reveal the valuable secrets we subconsciously hold. The understanding of spirit, in my opinion, is critical to all martial artists. We need to connect with it, understand it, and be able to draw from it when necessary.

I sincerely hope that this book stimulates you to further investigate the role that the teeth and jaws play in our ultimate survival and in the fulfillment of our individual destinies. It is our duty to break the shackles imposed by 'polite society'—which, in my opinion, are no less than a type of enforced castration—and make peace with this most basic of instincts that is necessary for our imminent survival. Martial artists who take the time to cultivate the chi of the teeth and jaws will simultaneously improve their fighting skills and overall health. And most importantly, we clear the path to our own self-realization and possibly grant ourselves the freedom to save our lives or the lives of those we love.

END BONUS BOOK
TEETH IN MORTAL COMBAT
How to Unleash Your Basic Instinct For Survival

Eat Like A Bird and Brush Your Beak.
A Simple Way To Prevent A Toothless Tweet.

—*from the TAO TE TOOTH*

Teeth in Mortal Combat

How To Unleash Your Basic Instinct For Survival

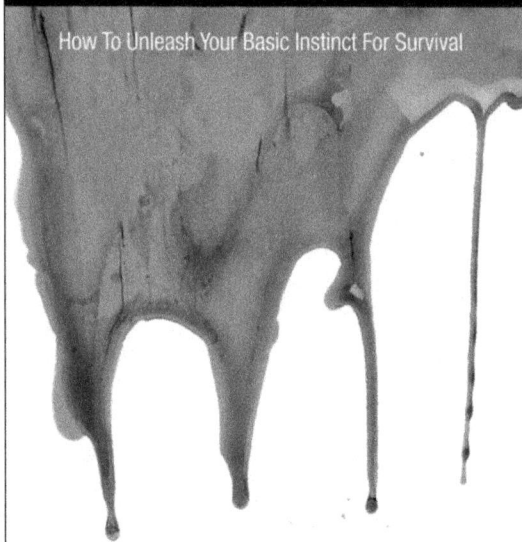

Lester Sawicki, DDS

TEETH
IN MORTAL
COMBAT

*Bonus Chapters
26 through 43*

CHAPTER 26
IMPROVE YOUR MARTIAL ARTS THROUGH...YOUR TEETH?

Improving your martial arts is not as hard as you might think when you cut out the "cr#p" and strip your training down to the basics. Most practitioners think that improving their martial arts means they have to sign-up for expensive one-of-a-kind "secret" training sold by World Champion Fighters. Others feel queasy about punching the lights out of their fellow students. And even worse, most people cringe when they think about getting "clobbered" by a weapon of mass destruction.

But it doesn't have to be like this. In fact, you can improve your martial arts without mortgaging your house, sparring with your neighbor's teenage brat, or suffering a steel-toe boot tattooed onto your chin.

It's as simple as a small twist in the way you think about your life and your basic instinct to survive. It's 100% accessible (not hidden) through my website and book, and I've proven to myself and other dedicated warriors that you WILL improve your martial arts, if you dare to... *Unleash Your Basic Instinct To Survive!*

I call it Teeth In Mortal Combat because sharp, strong, healthy teeth are considered the benchmark for the survival of any animal species, even before man (the greatest of warriors) fearlessly braved his territory.

And as you'll see on the following pages, it starts with the most critical awakening to the "real" world around you that your martial arts needs.

Let me help you "Unleash Your Most Basic Instinct To Survive," starting RIGHT NOW!

CHAPTER 27
NEVER GET CLOBBERED AGAIN!

To All Independent-Minded, Free-Thinkers who demand the truth, still love America, and love all the good things it stands for...
When your instinct is humming on all cylinders...
When your fighting skills are rock solid...
When your vital energy can zap an aggressor before he has a chance to blink...
That's when... you'll never get "clobbered" again

You're about to discover the revolutionary secret that can help your instinct get there.

Dear Martial Arts Friends,
This year you can...
 ✓ *Grapple with the best at your dojo—without hesitation...*
 ✓ *Visit other self-defense schools—without dodging challengers...*
 ✓ *And enter tournaments with a "King of the Hill" confidence...*

When your instinct is at the top of its game --
THERE'S NO REASON YOU SHOULD
GET YOUR CHOPS BUSTED

We all know that *'one person'* who never loses.

They can take on opponents all day long. They can spend their entire free time in dojos, boxing gyms, parks, and grimy schools...

But when you're *wiped, drained, bloody and raw* and look to them for some sympathy, all they can say is...

tough luck, but I don't ever lose my instincts…
… AND THEY'RE RIGHT!

What's their secret?
The SAME pit bull security system
waiting to be unleashed in YOU

Here's how you do it… *and in one moment I'll show you how easy it is…*

Think of society as a siege against your life force. If you're going to make it through without a single scar you must…

SECURE THE GATES with everything you've got! You have instinct—a protective barrier that is *designed to keep invaders out.* Don't leave it locked in a box…help your body release it to keep criminals OUT.

Order your internal warriors to fight back and fight HARD. If there's an opening, you're armed with *Natural Killer Instincts* that can spot it, strike vital spots, and disable any invader in seconds. Help your primitive instincts be as ruthless, skilled, and quick as they can be.

Expose hidden taboos! Criminals, aggressors, and opponents aren't the only dangers trying to sabotage your life force. Governments, cults, and society in general can chip away at it. A strong defensive instinct can handle all of them at once, but it needs to be freed from its cage. You have a responsibility to become aware of   society's hidden taboos. Supply the right training and help your instincts escape to freedom. Employ the best mental and energetic weapons to always stay alert to keep threats in check!

And here's the important part… **every living person is capable of sharpening their instinct… and now it's** *easier than ever.*

INSANE TIMES
Even Big Brother Admits Fraud
And Deception... Again!

The public has been warned for years of the dangers of fluoride in our drinking water by scientists both in the United States and Europe. But our local governments have forced it by fluoridating public water supplies. In 2005, eleven Environmental Protection Agency (EPA) Unions representing over 7000 EPA employees called for a moratorium on adding fluoride in the nation's drinking water. But municipalities, by the thousands, are still dumping the dangerous chemical into water supplies.

Cardiac by-pass surgery instead of common sense exercise and diet. Mass immunizations against viruses that are over-hyped and have no real threat to the average healthy person. Cell phone electromagnetic radiation and parotid tumors. Vioxx tragedies. Diabetes that can be naturally reversed, yet physicians still get their patients hooked on insulin injections.

The system appears to be crashing and the "bosses" appear to be stealing all they can in the guise of "our best interest." They are in charge and can care less about our real safety. Yes, the foxes are in charge of the hen house. We the people are pacified with media controlled propaganda.

Why do we swallow all this hypocrisy? The answer is that we the people don't know that we don't know. We are fed pacifism in our churches and the same in our schools and we never ask questions.

How can a minority government supported by corporate fat cats make a perpetual war on the majority citizens? The answer is that they have propaganda and they have the guns. And don't forget they have control over our money supply.

I cannot believe the downright disinterest of even the most "educated" people about how governments, big money and society in general enslave the whole world with their hoaxes and taboos.

Think now! The American people struggle to get an education, work their entire lives for a house they can call their own little bit of freedom on earth, yet they never so much as ask a question about the poisonous chemicals and drugs that are hidden in our food supply.

What is wrong with us? And if you're aware of the problem you might think there is no way to win a *"rigged game in a black hole"*—only grumbling and death writhing allowed.

We may be social animals with a desire to conform and force others to do so as well. We seem to be hard-wired to feel more secure if we huddle together in fear. The good news is that we are now experiencing history's most difficult evolutionary transformation and you are at the cutting edge of breaking free from the stranglehold of society.

**You Could be on the Verge of the
Most Devastating Meltdown
You Have EVER Seen!
AND...
It's your turn to fight back—
Discover the best way to break through taboos against
right acting and thinking and unlock your
BASIC INSTINCT FOR SURVIVAL**

It's an accepted belief, if you want self-confidence against opponents, you need your full instinct on guard 24 hours a day. One tiny inhibition (which can easily happen due to society's "rules") and uninvited aggressive behavior could be there to take advantage of you.

But until now, the only option you have is to fight back with one hand tied behind your back.

That won't do a thing!

Your instinct for self-defense is very simple—but it's incredible. In fact, an instinct with all cylinders firing should be able to destroy any invader. However, making sure your instinct is allowed "free will" to be in the right place, at the right time, in the right way is another issue—and I believe my book, *Teeth in Mortal Combat,* has an answer.

As in most cultures of the world, society gives us certain signals that tell us what to do, where to do it, and how to do it. By controlling and influencing these signals, institutions strangle your instinct's ability to deploy the plan of defense or attack that it knows best for the situation at hand. In a way your instinct is a well trained army that has been ordered to lay down their weapons. This way, if an intruder is lurking around the corner, your instinct won't automatically spring into action. It will be wasting time assembling the troops and support for the deployment of your most important lines of defense.

That's why you have to keep your instinct protected from negative influences. And if your instinct is already corrupted with a tightly wound internal virus, you have to uncoil and expunge it A.S.A.P.

Did you know that most martial arts teachers and Masters have NO IDEA why you're fighting skills are not improving? And that's a shame. **Because I've uncovered a surprising answer— your mouth and instinct!** And it has NOTHING to do with shouting "kiai."

The problem is martial artists aren't aware of the *"problem"* and their instincts aren't *juiced up.* Sure, you can be stimulated into boosting performance but then you're amped up only on command and usually after getting bashed. Your most basic instincts never kick in to explode into the ultimate fighting machine you truly are. And in my book you'll find answers to instinct awareness that are hiding right behind your two front teeth.

Flood Your Body With The Most Skill-Enhancing Martial Arts Discovery On Earth

When I discovered the shocking results of my intensive research   into the root causes of today's most common martial arts problems, I was literally stunned.

Suddenly, everything mainstream self-defense gurus thought about the causes of fighting arts problems was obsolete—as my investigations pointed to a brand-new, totally unexpected culprit…

TABOOS BY SOCIETY!

That's right! It may sound outlandish, but according to my research, society has a major role in your self-defense deficiencies. In fact, if you give my explosive discovery a tooth-fighting chance, you'll come to the same astonishing concision:

Every known weakness, from low self-esteem to shaky confidence, short attention span, foggy awareness, slow reaction time, disconnected intention, and more…come from the same root cause…Taboos. These problems are so widespread you could say it's an epidemic.

You could be suffering from taboo over!load!

My groundbreaking work concludes…

**"All mental and emotional blocks that interfere
with mastering a martial art are
rooted in the negative taboos society imposes on us."**

Taboos are so corrosively destructive that they are considered a seedbed for most, if not all, martial arts frustrations. In short: your consciousness may be soaking and drowning in an ocean of taboos—hook, bait, and sinker trolling you at the bottom—and they are destroying your life!

You don't have to be one of the bottom feeders!

**Nothing Good Happens When Each Mental Thought
Reflected in Every Organ, Tissue, and Cell
in Your Body is Soaking in Taboos!**

**<u>SHOCKER:</u>
Taboo Overload Makes You Want To Grab On To Even
More Taboos No Matter How Hard You Struggle In Life!**

And I believe that this little book can **REALLY Save Your Life!**
It's the **Ultimate Taboo Crusher** that Can **Lift Your Body and
Mind to a "Super Safety Zone"**

One your consciousness reaches the "zone"…you can enjoy some remarkable "Side Effects." And the simple discovery you're about to read about in my book may trigger a stunning turn-around that is nothing short of amazing. The sheer scope of possibilities you own is astounding. I wrote *Teeth in Mortal Combat* to help you combat the imbalances associated with living in today's society and to make sure that every aspect of your self-defense instinct is efficient and ready for "game time"... so you never have to worry about leaving your house naked.

And that's just a *tiny part* of the reason my book will help you blast through nonsensical taboos that lock you up. Just take a look at this...

First, your instinct has protective barriers, but they can be layered with taboo after taboo. Finally, the full weight of society's rules prevents the sleeping giant from being aroused.

Think of your teeth, tongue, and jaw as an ironclad gate, bridge, and gear protecting the entry into the castle of your body, heart and soul. Instinct is the driving force opening and closing your defense system. My book gives you a way to make sure the entrance to your fortress is as solid as a mountain... AND that your instinct guards the gate free of oppressive taboos... AND this is everyday 24/7 security—not just a boost in energy when it's too late and your defenses have been violated.

An aggressor would be foolish, crazy and nuts to take on ... a body surging with Primal Instinct!

I believe my book can help peel away generations of negative influences on your instinct. After reading it, you'll be more aware of how your teeth, tongue, and jaws can activate and enhance, with efficiency, the path to victory and self-realization.

Teeth in Mortal Combat is the one breakthrough book with the power to give you ultimate FREEDOM FROM FEAR. It has a powerhouse of revealing information that can:

A.) Boost your self-defense skills so that you can stay at the top of your game.

B.) Increase the strength of your teeth and jaws as your most basic and original line of defense... a solid wall of protection.

C.) Purify your energy to let loose a blurring wave of effortless, flowing, dynamic motion as efficient as possible by making you fast and ruthless...when you need it...using your most astounding weapon...instinct.

I feel very confident that if you put into action the principles in my book, you'll most likely never get caught off guard again. And with my 30 day purchase price guarantee you could soon be free of fear forever.

The information I reveal in my book is the greatest unexpected breakthrough I've ever seen.

Stop living in fear—You have a destiny to survive.
You must take steps _Right Now_
to safeguard your future and
Unleash your Instinct!

The Handwriting is on the Wall. You Can Either Bury Your Head in the Sand or Heed the Sober Warning—with real solutions—that My Book Gives You.

Hey, I'm honestly NOT trying to scare you. One of the reasons I wrote the book is because I believe there is a *solution* to all of this!

A solution for our country—and a solution for us as individuals.

But the solution will only make sense once you understand the cause and get a feel for the physical and mental exercises recommended.

Skeptical? I don't blame you. After all, this is news you won't hear from anyone in the mainstream media. And rest assured, the government, religious institutions, and big corporate controllers will remain very tight-lipped about it, too. Why? Because if this kind of news ever drifted down to the general public, *it would cost them elections and billions of dollars in profits!*

And only the <u>truth</u> will set you free.

The chilling truth revealed in the book will hopefully help you see the significance of "true freedom" before it's Too Late and everything around you collapses...

**...but you're still standing strong, solid
and NOT Stupid!**

When you look around and see all the problems occurring now—how they are ultimately being caused by the fact that society is choking back our instincts...the you also see a big, big part of the solution.

A society can only do what we are witnessing—self-destruct, because the longer and thicker a leash it extends—the more it loses control. It is like a cancer that eats its host from within. Yet history has taught us that it's the aware and instinct driven individual that survives even the hardest of times. And the truest survival is found in breaking all negative taboos laid upon us by society.

You see, there's so much more I want to tell you about this exclusive new book and I realized that my message was simply far too urgent and valuable not to share with anyone who'd listen. So I strongly urge you to get a copy to carry it with you and share it with your friends as I'm sharing it with you.

Believe me, at a time in America when the stakes are unbelievably high—when your life and complete well being are at risk—you NEED accurate, unbiased information.

You need the TRUTH. And in my book, Teeth In Mortal Combat, the truth behind today's biggest health and wealth lies and half-truths that mainstream media is feeding us can be uncovered by unleashing your basic instinct to survive.

From risky, unnecessary medical procedures... all the way to the many blatant lies being spoon fed to us by the fat cats on Wall Street... it's time to stop blindly accepting what we are being told.

And I learned the hard way from my own research... the basic instinct to survive is the most trusted source you can rely on and the best way to live for an enriched life... safer, happier, healthier.

Now I want the same for you!

Join Me as I Blow the Whistle on the "controllers"
In Power—So You Can Protect Health and Welfare
for Yourself and Your Loved Ones in the Years to Come!

Chapter 28
ARE YOU DOOMED TO FALL?

News shocker:

**Without this simple understanding,
all martial artists are doomed to fail.**

Training manuals and ancient esoteric texts don't have it, but my breakthrough book does!

**A MIRACLE?
Not Even Close, But
This One Simple Secret
Cuts Right To The Quick For
Unbelievable Results!**

Guaranteed to give you amazing insight—or your money back!
"I was in great mental anguish, but this really worked. The results were so astonishing!"
"It opened up my eyes and blew my mind…freed me from decades of misguided advice."
"The reports don't lie. I was stunned by this discovery…"
"My training made a quantum leap once I busted the chains."

My research shows:
**Your martial arts isn't working to your expectations
because it may not be blasting through
the source of your demons**

If your martial arts skills aren't improving…If some visualizations work for you some of the time, but none give you pure

100% results, _Teeth In Mortal Combat_ could change your life.

After many years of martial arts research, I believe I've finally discovered why so many systems fall so short in giving you the satisfaction of accomplishment you deserve. The reason: Too often...

The training goes after the wrong target!

Many of today's most popular fighting arts schools are designed to teach ancient, Eastern traditional systems of education and indoctrination. Others Westernize the training and philosophy. But none of them target what may actually be at the root of your disappointment: social taboos.

A taboo is a moral or cautionary restriction placed upon certain actions by authorities which if ignored will result in specific negative consequences. Because of the fear instilled at a young age of indoctrination, societal taboos are so well accepted in our world that they almost seem natural, correct, and necessary.

Here's how it works: An authority senses a threat to his/her power—it can be as minor as a small bump during play, or even just a sudden glare from you when he demands taxes for the land your family has farmed for many generations—and he reacts by:

1.) **Sending his henchmen** to intimidate you for the bump or glare.
2.) **Proclaiming Taboos** to essentially prevent you from bumping or glaring again.

After several generations of taboos, freedom of expression is broken, hard feelings subside, and everything seems normal. But sometimes things go badly...

Sometimes we take the taboo too seriously and our body and mind fail to steer around it. So like a gear that's stuck in a position, the taboo continues to block our energy beyond our means of adapting. All too often, the taboos block our natural flow of life energy and we're soon beset with illness, disease, bad luck, and a general dissatisfaction with living.

Plus, as we age, the socially accepted taboo can become as difficult to remove as an indelible tattoo. Meanwhile, you keep busting your brains trying to figure a way to make living bearable and profitable again. But it's like mapping a route to Mars with a toy compass.

In this case, all the hours in your dojo…the daily workout… stringent diet…focused meditation…mantra…prayer…affirmation…psycho-therapy…self-help books…etc. won't work if they can't get through to that one taboo which is choking your free energy channel.

NOW, I BELIEVE THE DISCOVERY REVEALED IN MY BOOK CAN BUST THROUGH ANY TABOO, SURGICAL-LY EXPOSE THE SOURCE AND FREE YOUR LIFE FROM THE TORTUROUS RACK OF MENTAL CONDITIONING IMPOSED BY OPPRESSIVE AUTHORITIES.

Taboos are normally dissolved by living in harmony with nature away from society. But most people today, living in a world of more than 6 billion, have completely lost touch with nature. In fact, if they tried to return to nature they would surely be putting their life in danger. So the taboos remain, and they end up with torturing piercing mental anguish.

Now, I've discovered a way using common martial arts training techniques that I believe can boot out the taboo that is holding you back. It's all revealed in my book. It works for me and I know it will work for you!

The problem began when you were an infant and it's about to end when you buy my book.

It took me, afflicted with the same mental pain you're having, years of research to finally discover…

A <u>solution</u> to the nightmarish agony of living in a world without much hope of personal fulfillment in my martial arts and personal life.

Most friends, teachers, and professional advisors will often tell you that what you need is an attitude adjustment through short personal time off away from your normal living and work environment. Of course, you know as I learned that means no cure, no relief.

Now, there's new hope for people like you.

And the solution is clearly explained in both my book, Teeth In Mortal Combat and the training video in this website. I searched for years spending thousands of dollars on solutions when the "Aha" moment finally came. And the answer, hard to believe, isn't right in front of your nose but right BEHIND your nose within your oral cavity—teeth, tongue, jaws, AND brain!

The taboos involve your most basic life support—your mouth: eating, drinking, talking, breathing, AND fighting.

I believe I found the answer and immediately sought to share it with the world. In fact, I believe it is a moral imperative that what's uncovered in my book be shared with the rest of the world and most importantly, the martial arts community.

What you'll learn is a very effective technique to crack away the hard barrier of society's taboos, and free your body and mind from their excruciating hold—allowing you to release your true inner expression and live life with no holds barred! Completely on track to self-realization! Totally!

That's what my book does, and that's why you shouldn't go another day without taking my challenge to try it!

Relieve The Constrictions In Your Energy
So You Can Enjoy Your Usual Daily Routine
Proven Effective For Me and I'm Confident You Will Get
Similar Results

I Rank It #1 For Effectiveness

If you don't remove the taboo, you don't remove the bitterness.
Life's Greatest Pleasure Is Doing What People Say
You Cannot Do

Powerfully Effective For Martial Artists

"My martial arts training wasn't 'better,' it was
supercharged on steroids!"

CHAPTER 29
GO BEYOND ORDINARY TRAINING METHODS

*Teeth In Mortal Comba*t **Takes You Beyond Ordinary Training Methods to Results You Can Feel!**

Thousands of Americans Are Now Using this Breakthrough Discovery to Help Fight Their Lack of Self-Confidence, Low Self-Esteem, and Decision Making Problems, Shaking Mainstream Establishments to the Core!

Now, you may ask, how? The answer lies within the specific research and rare revelations that make up this powerful book. These essential elements are not found in the front pages of your daily newspaper, best seller lists, training manuals, martial arts schools, and yellowing pages of legendary Asian texts. We wish we had this knowledge years ago!

An overwhelming amount of positive news has been accumulating that proves the effectiveness of all the principles clearly laid out in the book. Much more effective than years of misguided meditation, it may prevent the wrong reactions before an unexpected personal attack occurs or the competitive environment of a tournament psyches you out.

This Mind Bending Discovery Can Save You From An Unnecessary Death Sentence

The book unfolds a combination of theories that unify us with Mother Earth and are capable to transform the lives of tens of thousands of people. These ideas include vital messages that are essential for a healthy body and provide nourishment for a free spirit.

Teeth In Mortal Combat has been customized to transform illogical and inhibiting taboos, never openly discussed before, into a flurry of potent punches thrusting you forward to give you the best chance to break through all prior mental limitations until victory is achieved. That's why the book has been recognized to give you back the life of excellence you desire—where **Miracles Are Accomplished...**

It's SO easy! Even if you have NOT been training martial arts for self-defense, it's not too late to turn your life around. This book can hap get you back on the road to self-determination almost immediately. Start now and keep your instincts performing at peak efficiency for the rest of your life.

The moment you begin reading this new emancipating book, the common sense conclusions enter your consciousness immediately with an energy explosion your body has never experienced. They go to work at once without fail and begin balancing your energy system so you can feel fast results, because these ideas are absorbed directly into your DNA and go where needed most. It is absolutely astonishing!

**Save Yourself from Overbearing Institutions
and Unrestricted Government Control,
and Don't Let Your Destiny Be Deprived of
the Freedom to Express Its Rich Future**

With the cutting edge principles of *Teeth In Mortal Combat,* you can prove to yourself how to keep your basic instincts for survival healthy and repair any damage already done. It can help protect your precious life by increasing the circulation of inherited signals at a more invigorating level. Changing the way you think about society's rules provide better spiritual nourishment to your imagination and even affects the tiniest brain cells physically. You will know firsthand how vibrant and revitalized this book can make you—no matter your past negative habits!

This Amazing Book Can Help Restore A Strong Healthy Mind Set...With Clear Instincts

CHAPTER 30
THE DUMB AND DANGEROUS MISTAKE

The Dumb & Dangerous
SELF-DEFENSE MISTAKE
Instructors Make Everyday

It's their mistake ... but it's you to blame!

How to fix what instructors miss ...
so you can stop the blame and take responsibility now!

**Forget everything
you've been told about
DISARMING YOUR ATTACKER
... It's Nonsense**

The real reason you're not getting the consistent results you need is because many teachers have it ALL WRONG.

Your limbs may ache, burn, and quiver, but it's actually NOT YOUR BODY interfering with your progress.

Thanks to a surprising discovery I made pursuing a career as a dentist while studying both martial arts and meditation, the REAL CULPRIT OF DEFEAT has been uncovered ...

**... And I expect thousands will soon report an answer
to their sorry martial arts skills, as I did!**

I'll never forget my hard working friends and acquaintances whose lives were almost destroyed by their obsession to master a fighting art. I, myself, had no better luck and it was heart-breaking to see dedicated students depressed with all hope for success fading.

We all tried expensive seminars, obscure meditation techniques, and even psychics. Sure, we learned something with value but our mental book of knowledge seemed to weigh down our "real" progress even more.

Then one day, after experimenting with my dreams, I suddenly discovered the power of teeth, tongue and jaws. And thank God I did! Switches started to turn on, dominoes began to tumble, and I finally found something that truly and consistently worked for me. My feelings and instincts began to talk to me, with good and dependable insights.

So why did these simple techniques work so well when *everything else* failed?

Because as soon as I began to repair the critical, but overlooked culprits that were really causing the blocks in my energy-instinct flow, unchecked negative signals embedded by a controlling society began to dissolve away.

And when you mix the free spirit of martial arts with the senseless and limiting taboos of society, it's like kindling for a red hot fire! The aching and burning of emotional turmoil can be relentless.

Then the depression settles in and you can say goodbye to any progress in your chosen art. It's a downward spiral that can wreck your quality of life, month after month, year after year. And thousands of martial artists keep suffering needlessly. But just like me, you don't have to anymore!

I'm breaking free from the chains of society— *you can too!*

In my more than 25 years as a dentist and martial arts researcher, I've never known any training method that comes close to the speed, effectiveness, and safety of Teeth In Mortal Combat. When I first discovered it I knew I had to share this with the martial arts community. It literally blew me away! Hard core results proven time and time again as I practiced daily.

The Secret Behind the Breakthrough…

Two "cutting-edge" tools that work
together to stop the real causes of every
struggling martial artist's frustration!

Teeth + Imagination

For the first time ever, I've combined the power of teeth and mind into a method that breaks the chains of slavery that society straps you with from a very young age. Together they crack open a doorway to "real" freedom that other training methods simply miss.

The Result?

…A true breakthrough that can improve the lives of thousands of martial artists suffering from all forms of mental anguish because of lack of progress.

I did it…

NOW IT'S YOUR TURN!

I urge you to read my book, *Teeth In Mortal Combat,* and please forget everything you've ever been told about disarming your attacker.

BUY IT NOW!

Seriously, do you know any martial artist who after 5, 10, or 25 years is having a tough time of it and says, "Yep, the old habits are gone, I'm feeling great about my level of skill, and I'll become a Master within the next 18 months." It just doesn't happen. What you usually hear is, "Looks like my dreams were greater than my ability," or "Heading to another expensive weekend seminar for my next injection of chi. I hope it sticks this time."

The conventional fighting arts approach for training self-defense is a complete and shameful failure for the average Joe. *It does not work.* And there are few good choices.

Most martial arts schools apply a grim superficial approach that ignores the real cause of your stagnant chi-instinct and simply attempt to smother your symptoms. What you often wind up with is another set of problems that are even worse. You're left to believe that you'll have to deal with your dissatisfaction day in and day out until your meridians are cleansed. There may be some truth to that, but **that's no way to live.** And now you don't have to.

Finally, a better way to restore your enthusiasm

You really do have better choices—ways to actually address the causes of your growing frustrations. And you can read more about them in this website and in my book, which some readers consider…

…A Bright New Light for Martial Artists

…and a Godsend for thousands of dedicated fighting arts practitioners that have all but given up on their goal. It worked for me..

…It can work for you, too!

Teeth In Mortal Combat
**Can Show You How To
Unleash Your Basic Instinct To Survive!**

**Refresh Your Instinct
Save Your Independence**

Your heart can be in great shape. You can be disease free. Your mind can be sharp as a tack. Your bones and joints can be strong. But when your instinct fails, your quality of life could quickly be reduced to one you wouldn't wish on your worst enemy.

*Society's rules and regulations impair instinct reaction
and they are one of the top causes of loss of independence.*

So, it's no surprise that there are lots of products and seminars on the market that claim to help your self-determination.But here's the problem: most of them are filled with advice that you simply cannot incorporate into your physical training. and get this: some of them actually add to the problem.

This really bothers me. With thousands seeking solutions to improve their connection with the "force", with thousands doing all they can to preserve their precious independence to live life to it's fullest, I saw that most of them were wasting their money on products and seminars that don't have a snowball's chance in hell of breaking the stifling chains of society.

So I did something about it. I wrote the book based on my personal discoveries that show how the four pillars of teeth, tongue, jaws, and mind can be beneficial to your health, martial arts, and freedom to live as you choose.

Teeth In Mortal Combat concentrates into one book my training secrets with all the essential coordinates you need to create a map for the biggest "jail break" of your life. A carefully laid

254 Teeth In Mortal Combat — *Bonus Chapters*

out plan that helps you break free of deeply embedded negative mental code placed there by a society of "software" developers with questionable motives. And it is the ONLY book I know of that does this!

The book has only one purpose: to help you stop wasting your time and money on "fluff" and get down to the business of "gruff."

Your Instinct Is Starving for Attention

Feed it what it needs and LIKE MAGIC it can help you go through life with:

> Added confidence
>
> No second guessing
>
> No self-doubt
>
> No flip-flopping decisions
>
> No fear of what's behind the curve

Like every other part of your body, your energy-instinct requires special attention. Without it, your freedom of expression eventually starves and shuts down. When you feed your basic instinct to survive, it keeps working. And if you feed it, you better be able to chew it thoroughly. The theory is pretty much that simple.

So naturally, I discovered and strongly believe that every martial arts training program should focus on the teeth, tongue, jaws and mind to give you the most basic element of surviving in a nasty world. Regain control over your life and become bulletproof against the relentless bombardment of a host of societal and environmental factors that unleash destructive forces onto your sensitive energies.

Just so happens, it takes years for the bombardment to take its toll on us. And that's why we're all used to it and don't even notice it taking over our lives.

But does my new discovery mean you have to go around wearing scamming-scanning goggles all the time to protect yourself from a world of unfriendly elements? It wouldn't hurt. But it won't do much to improve your instinct to survive ... not to mention your handsome looks.

I believe Teeth In Mortal Combat is the better way to deflect those stealth bombers set loose by the real war of terror. And I believe it can come to your rescue, allowing you to see the light through the darkness, so you can hit your target goal in life with war-winning accuracy. That's how effective I believe my book is and reports from readers are coming back supporting my stand.

My book is the ONLY BOOK that has an answer that you can put to work—day one—with practical training advice that fights off the yoke around your throat. In other words, it strengthens your self-determination so you don't bleed to death losing your energy and expression of free will. And make no mistake. You don't want any chi leaking from your self-defense pipeline.

My book has been shown to serve as an anti-terrorist agent, keeping your energy running freely and your instinct for survival healthy.

How Much Would You Pay for a Lifetime of Healthy Instinct?

Ask a martial artist suffering another bout of depression that same question.

Look, I believe my book is such an amazing revelation that I don't want anything to keep it away from you. If you cut up your credit cards and can't buy online with electronic payment, just send a check or money order.

This is your chance. Without risk! See for yourself why I'm so excited about it.

Fair enough?

Then BUY IT NOW!

Tell me you want to Unleash Your Basic Instinct To Survive. The fastest, easiest, safest way to protect your path to glory and enjoy winning, in every way, for life!

You have nothing to lose, except your independence, if you choose not to look after your instinct.

Looking out for you,

Lester Sawicki, D.D.S

Chapter 31
DON'T BECOME A FITNESS FRUITCAKE

**Now that it's a multi-billion-dollar industry,
the snake-oil shysters are crawling out of the woodwork,
intent on making you their next
FITNESS FRUITCAKE**

Psychologists may not help you. Trainers in fitness clubs often think only the most expensive exercise equipment is the best. Your work-out video is likely to do little more than read the script back to you—but the script in videos can be misleading—and in some cases, downright wrong.

Is it any wonder that millions of fitness seekers are still suffering from lack of focus, mindful intention, and generally diminished instinct driven success.

Don't you dare let them ruin your body/mind connection.
Arm yourself with the newest discovery that spells out exactly how you could maximize the health benefits you actually need ... vital physical, mental and natural instinct driven reflexes with a strong fighting mind.

Millions of fitness fanatics are strapped into $200 running shoes and zipped up designer hooded sweats, forgetting where their keys are or not confident about making good, solid, spur of the moment decisions.

Men and women from coast to coast are pumping slow burns, running, stretching, sweating, balancing and twisting yoga poses

Fitness books and videos are flying off the shelves of holistic retail outlets; however, those concerned with their natural born instincts might still have reason to worry.

I'm concerned, my friend.

People are working out more than ever before, yet they're energy driven instincts not fully unleashed the way nature intended, are diminishing in every way. Only a small handful of men and women are enjoying the full benefits promised.

Meditation could help you prevent—even reverse—those serious free flowing energy problems and many others. Science proves it! Ironically, it is because of the near-miracle benefits of meditation that the marketing of fitness for longevity has turned into a multi-billion-dollar industry—an enterprise that's usually motivated by greed.

And the shysters are creeping out of the woodwork to get a piece of the action. Junk seminars and classes abound. Websites are selling improbable dreams with hyped-up claims, robbing you of the improved life you seek.

Which specific visualizations and exercises should you be practicing? And which ones should you avoid?

Sadly, your fitness trainer and guru may not tell you. Your spiritual advisor probably can't either. And you can forget about the federal government. I doubt they'd want you to know anything about powerful mental self-development, or anything else that competes with their hidden agenda of world domination.

<u>BUT I WANT YOU TO KNOW.</u> And I'm going to help you cut through all the confusion and tell you—in plain English—how you could break the chains of control society shackled you with, in order to achieve success and satisfaction in every part of your life … energetic and physical.

Every page of my incredible book gives you critical insights that are vital to your health and well-being. In plain English, my book in your hands slashes away the binding ropes you innocently let society wrap around your struggling arms, legs, torso and neck.

And if you're in great health with strong heart and muscles you might wonder what Teeth in Mortal Combat can do for you. Sadly, people like you often don't know what they're missing until a bus hits them as they cross the street. It's alarming but true. You could think you're bullet-proof but, unfortunately, life's experience hasn't tested you thoroughly. You're likely looking at yourself with blurred eyes and lacking true objective self-analysis.

Stop being fooled! Buy my book and let it's clearing light shine through the misty veil of confusion society drapes over you. I feel very certain the information and theories I present can help protect you from becoming another fitness fruitcake. I have no hidden agenda. The information I give you is pure and proven to myself, strictly objective and tested with years of personal experience. I'm not selling you hype and have only one purpose...

To help YOU!
Avoid the Hidden Dangers
Nobody's Telling You About

If you're about to reverse a lifetime of inhibitions holding you back by acting out the popular slogan "just do it", for instance, you could be damaging your kidney energy.

If you're trying to figure out through mainstream media the main impetus behind government policy, you could be draining the power of your spleen.

You won't find these warnings in martial arts books or painted scrolls hanging on the walls of your dojo.

It's alarming, but true. You could be bleeding corn dogs, thinking it's the proper amount of exercise with mental conditioning and still be wondering why you're not feeling the promised benefits.

Stop for a moment and stand back. I want to help you "get it." And I want to keep you out of harm's way by revealing to you the littlest-known danger—the lost connection with your teeth, tongue and jaws.

What are the teeth, tongue and jaws, exactly? Where do they come from? What do they do in your body? How are they related with the energy centers of the body and do they really connect with the flow of chi through the teeth meridians? These are basic questions that far too few martial artists—even those who have been studying chi for years—can answer.

But all those questions and many more are addressed in my book. This book is packed with valuable information on self-defense and the pure art of living FREE! No more roaming up and down the aisles of book stores in search of what you need to take you to the next level of excellence. After reading this book you'll know. And you'll know much more than your teacher, I assure you. You'll be armed with the key that unlocks the most basic information you need to know about surviving and thriving in a world that seems to be splintering apart more and more of your freedoms.

Well, you don't have to live like that anymore. It's time to reveal the best-kept secret for peace and well-being. How to allow your energy to regulate and control what gets into your emotional crystal palace and what attaches to the precious jewels within.

Of course, there's no way for me to know exactly what personal concerns are troubling you right now. But I can tell you that you will discover a helpful remedy you can use on a daily basis. And as you'll see after reading the first few pages, I don't beat around the bush with warm fuzzy ancient aphorisms.

From the very first sentence right through to the very last, the focus is on YOU and my latest research breakthroughs that could help you regain control and add productive years to your life.

And so it is with pure intentions and motives that I bring you right now...

Teeth In Mortal Combat
How To Unleash Your Basic Instinct For Survival

When your chi instinct is in control, life is good: effective life systems prevail. When your instinct is lacking free flow, a state of confusion often results: an unhealthy condition of imbalance and disorganized flow of events.

My book offers a rescue plan for people like you that want to take back control of their life without the limitations imposed by society. It shows you ways to adjust your mindset and eventually get back to feeling comfortable inside. The methods revealed work for me and, if you give them a chance, I guarantee they'll work for you too!

Chapter 32
NOT SEEN IN WORLD NEWS HEADLINES

The Amazing New Findings Inside
TEETH IN MORTAL COMBAT
Were Likely Buried And Lost In
A Hidden Ancient Chinese Tomb.

Now, you can be the first to have express access to Forbidden Martial Arts Secrets HUSHED-UP by Masters of World Domination. Some Fighting Arts Insiders **gasped in disbelief**, but the results speak for themselves…and **would rock the world—if anyone saw them!**

Astonished Scientists Discover and Prove Beyond Any Doubt:

Brain Damage PREVENTED…by NOT wearing football helmets?

Mouth Guards Make You Slower, Weaker, and Smaller?

Primitive Man, With Better Brain Fitness and Physical Fitness, Was Far Superior to Today's Puny "World's Strongest and Fastest"

Exercising Teeth and Jaws increases our ability to concentrate and complete mental tasks by up to 20% MORE!

Behind The Locked Gates of Your Dojo
What?! and WHY?! Did They "Forget" To Tell You?

Give Your Respect to Rock Solid Science:

Teeth Qi Kung produces saliva which releases a surge of insulin. Our body gets ready for a meal—JUST LIKE A TIGER!—insulin increases heart rate and sends at least 25-40 percent more blood to the brain. This gives our brain a blast of glucose and oxygen which helps us to think faster, respond stronger... AND protect and defend like a ruthless wild beast.

Teeth In Mortal Combat May Be The
Cure for "Brain Fitness + Physical Fitness"
You Never Heard About!

NOTE: The cures and hushed secrets revealed in this book are so shocking, you may wonder if they're exaggerated. *Actually, they may even be understated!* And when these discoveries become common knowledge, the *fat cats* that wave their clubs of power over us will start spending desperate billions to frantically cover up these *"dangerous"* threats to their kingdom. There's only one life-or-death question left to ask: "How long before this book is banned from the marketplace?"

Well, you don't have to worry... for now... because Pandora's Box has been opened... and an unstoppable force escaped... like miniature nuclear missiles... rocketing life-changing truths to all parts of the globe. And you are about to be hit head-on target with gut-breaking miracle solutions that exceed your wildest dreams.

Teeth In Mortal **Combat Wins With "Aces"**
too bad...
ALL MAJOR WARS
FOR WORLD DOMINATION FLUNK

Teeth In Mortal Combat leaves no wiggle room for giant mega-corporations, abusive government, and fanatic religious institutions trying to smother, with taboos, your instinct for freedom and survival. Inside the book you'll find theories that answer your most pressing physical and emotional needs. This is SO HOT, it makes nuclear fusion on the sun look like a toasted marshmallow.

And when the book convinces you, *beyond a shadow of all doubt,* the true value in preserving ALL your teeth (free of tooth decay and gum disease), your "Holistic" Dentist should become your best friend.

Please let me clarify: I'm not condemning mainstream conventional dentistry. Some of the most skilled dental surgeons and specialists in all fields of dentistry are my best friends and I unhesitatingly refer my E.R. trauma patients to them. Especially the ones suffering severe infections, irascible diseases, and genetic and epigenetic disabilities. Patients that fit into these categories usually become civilian casualties in the typical modern battleground between corporate greed's no holds barred take-all-we-can deceptive advertising and the average American's weakened will power.

And this is where we need Special Forces to intervene and perform life saving battleground surgery. Dental specialists are Super Heroes with formally trained superior technical and artistic skills needed to arrest and correct near death conditions of tooth and body. A failed tooth and body can take only so much damage before its detox pathways become permanently clogged. That's where the surgeon comes in to cut out, burn, and carefully dispose the trash—saving your life—and if you don't have insurance you might be lucky to buy yourself a second chance at a healthier life.

But sooner or later…

if you want to thrive and survive…

you have to visit your Holistic Dentist and have a Spoonful of his Energized Super-Food. Because Holistic Dentistry is where you can find cures you never heard about—for free! These cures are documented and verified by mainstream doctors and dentists but hushed-up by yesterday's health establishment.

And this is where *Teeth In Mortal Combat* terrifies the 'good old buddies' network of controlling medical police that do all the 'hushing'. Why take risky and pricey medications when organic food, pure unadulterated water, and sun freshened air is your best medicine...and almost free? Just say, "NO!" Take a stand for yourself...and if you can't find the guts to do it...your best prescription for a recharged, pumped up spunk and toughness is... *Teeth In Mortal Combat*. This is the only book that shows you how to give yourself a shot in the arm of will power...the best vaccine against any threat to your freedom to live by instinct. And you'll be shocked when you read why the abundant power of the teeth, tongue and jaws are the prime ingredients of the vaccine...and this secret has been buried by the mainstream establishment for eons...and even your Holistic Dentist might not know this...but it's not his fault because the power of controlling "dark forces" is permeating everywhere.

So...isn't it time to do something in YOUR best interest?

STAND TALL AND NAKED IN THE SUN
SHOUT OUT LOUD TO THE WORLD
"I'M NOT GOING TO TAKE IT ANYMORE!"

...and scrub yourself clean of all negative thoughts and interferences you inherited from family and society...

UNLEASH YOUR INSTINCT FOR SURVIVAL

Buy the book, NOW!

Chapter 33
INSTINCT FREEZE

Read this now if you don't want
INSTINCT FREEZE

Dear Lovers of Free Style Living and Fighting,

You know how drinking a real-real cold slurpee can give you Brain Freeze? And how drugs cause Brain Fog? And a low level of vitamin "O" - oxygen - can lead to Brain Death?

Now, the most important book to hit the book stores, *Teeth In Mortal Combat*, is sending shock waves through the Martial Arts Community by flat out punching the lights out of tired and worn fighting techniques that "fake" the refinement of your instinct. Millions of martial artists throughout the world are getting scammed by sub-quality training manuals and this starts my teeth grinding!

Your instinct can suffer the same brain dementia that cripples so many seniors today. The problem starts with Instinct Freeze, turns into Fog, and if you do NOTHING, the end is DEATH. And youth has no real advantage nor resistance to this hidden epidemic. But if you're over 50, watch out! The damage might be irreversible, UNLESS...you read about and take the antidote clearly explained in the book.

Are YOU worried about clogged arteries, memory loss, Alzheimier's plaques, depression, dizziness, balance problems, weakness, confusion...? All of these... *and more*... are signs of Instinct Freeze and/or Fog. Your instinct for survival is chained up in a dark room and the mass media, controlled by mega billionaire power barons, is mostly responsible. And if you're like most people, either you're not aware of the problem or you don't know how to reverse it.

But that's all changing now because the breakthrough book, *Teeth In Mortal Combat,* is brewing up a major storm that could wipe out all negative influences in your life, reducing empires built on mind control to dust ... and it's starting to happen now. The Powers that Be know it's coming and they're desperately scrambling to prevent it. They're terrified of losing billions of profits and their control over you and your sacred instinct for survival, and are willing to do anything ... *anything* to sidestep their coming Armageddon.

And while most people sit passively on the sidelines, watching and listening for their own death knoll, I've discovered a way to take back control ... something so powerful, in fact, that even I was surprised what gains could be made! That's why I wrote *Teeth In Mortal Combat.* So both you and I can survive the escalating turmoil in our lives and the world we live in. But in order to do that, we have to first have some idea of what Instinct Freeze is, recognize it in our own life, and understand how it transformed into an uncomfortable constant Fog ... before ... Death Do Us Part.

Isn't it time to bolster your natural defenses—and fast? Live a life where the good times are rolling? Become the roaring tiger you were meant to be, rather than a helpless vegetable stumbling on celery stick legs. Then you better act quick, because the "dark forces" sucking up your life energy are getting more powerful with each day you procrastinate finding your solution and putting into play an action plan for survival.

Teeth In Mortal Combat Craters the Competition for Your Life Force...

...with a remedy that's been kept from you for ages. Most martial arts instructors are clueless...they keep feeding you expensive programs that give you some physical ability, but does nothing for your faltering instinct for survival. My book, at less than one-tenth of a penny per word, is without question much more effective than endless hours in the gym or dojo. But you've been kept in the dark, my friend, far too long.

The Holy Grail of Self-Defense and Self-Realization

I say it's time to break the silence. Your health and well-being are far too important to fall victim to silence. I am on a mission to open your eyes and ears so you too may benefit. Buy the book, read it, and then you can decide for yourself, if what I have to say make sense to you.

1.) Society has many taboos which they say are for your benefit, and many times, if not always, the side effects are worse than the social condition they are trying to correct.

2.) Most organizations are intended to suppress your ability to live freely and fulfill your visionary dreams.

3.) Profit-hungry companies are mainly interested in their profit—not yours.

Once Thought "Hopeless"
Now You Can Speak Up
and
Act Out

And I'm on your side. You'll be surprised, too, with the same results that surprised me! In the United States, where the influence of big corporate "con-gloms" has its strongest grip, the success I experienced sharpening my survival instincts cannot be ignored.

You need not stay in the dark any longer. Buy the book and shake free of taboos that emotionally and physically bind you prisoner from your innate ability to make miracles happen in your life. You'll find the ideas revealed fascinating and powerful. The book is indispensable for men and women of all ages. Schools and workplaces should pass it out *like throat lozenges!*

But you've got to act NOW because if you are teetering on the edge of Instinct Fog, it can become permanent if you don't do something immediately! The book is an indispensable guide for anyone seeking an end to a confused life filled with disappointments and tough decisions to make, no matter where you live. Even if you live in a small town or a remote area, you can find the help you need in the enlightening pages of the book.

Teeth In Mortal Combat is:

BIG

BEST

EXTREME

THE ULTIMATE

YOUR BEST FRIEND

FILLED WITH ANSWERS

RATED 5 STAR NUMBER ONE

THE END ALL OF DEADLY TABOOS

A LIFESAVER COMING OUT OF THE DARK

THE WORLD'S MOST ASTONISHING DISCOVERY

SIGNIFICANTLY BOOSTS JAWBONE MINERAL DENSITY

GOING BALLISTIC ON A SEARCH AND DESTROY MISSION

"BULLET PROOF" PROTECTION FOR YOUR KIDNEY ENERGY

A FORBIDDEN "TOOTH" MIRACLE THAT COULD SAVE YOUR LIFE

THE NEW "BULLY" ON THE BLOCK FIGHTING HARD FOR YOUR RIGHTS

SO HOT, THE FAT CATS THAT RULE THE WORLD ARE TRYING TO HUSH IT UP

Chapter 34
LONGEVITY TAI CHI IS IN THE TEETH

Longevity Tai Chi
Why settle for slow, soft, smooth Tai Chi at 90 years of age...
when you can

**Rejuvenate every aspect of youthing
with an explosive and exhilarating fierce Tai Chi dance
at a delightful 125 years of age!**

Dear Tai Chi Enthusiast,

Mark my words: This new breakthrough WILL change your Tai Chi goals as you know them today, <u>forever</u>. And I'm not talking about just another style of Tai Chi. This discovery—made recently—goes *light years* beyond all those notions, potions, and motions they sell as silly Tai Chi at hundreds of classes and seminars across the nation.

You see, longevity isn't just about slowing down and smoothing out your 108 forms. It's about keeping your vigor and vitality vibrant with volcanic fury well into your 100's.

And all those beauteous floating Tai Chi dreams are nothing more than last ditch efforts to offset the <u>effects</u> of time and gravity.

To TRULY *reclaim your youth* you must target what emerging research shows are the very causes of aging <u>**inside your body**</u>.

And this groundbreaking discovery doesn't just target those causes...It works to grapple them to a *screeching halt*...and then goes to work reinvigorating your whole body, from the inside out.

Which means you won't just look relaxed and powerful <u>in slow motion</u>...You may be able to **rewind the energy inside**

your cells to a time when furious fist play radiated from your childhood memories.

That's why I'm so certain that this brand-new approach to longevity will

Revolutionize the way you
restore childlike play into your Tai Chi—*and your life*.

Most of the "experts" will tell you that aging is one of the reasons martial artists switch from fast-hard to slow-soft styles.

But the misconception of "aging" is being rejected by modern science and research. The very process of safeguarding your health—and your youth…transforming it into an age-defying head-to-toe EVERYTHING-YOU-NEED Anti-Aging Powerhouse is no longer quantified a miracle in progress.

That's right—unless you're a relentless footballer or marathon runner with worn out hip sockets and knees or a weathered martial arts fighter with stiff broken knuckles—you can realistically and completely **rejuvenate your body and every cell**—*to run at peak performance*…a new you 30 years younger.

If you're serious about *changing the very course of your health and well being* and taking control of how your whole body responds to the effects of time, then **this is information you can't afford to be without.**

You'll feel *energized and renewed*…Ready to greet each day, knowing that your Tai Chi is stronger—and more PLAYFUL— than practitioners half your age…That your focus is **sharp as a pencil point** and have no trouble reacting to the changing circumstances…And that your quickness, speed and stamina hasn't lost the spark you had as a young stallion. Your body systems will be *primed for battle* against the many causes of aging.

If that's the sort of change you've been eager to see—**and feel**—in yourself, then the whole-body benefits of my exclusive breakthrough will be, quite frankly, priceless.

And you could start getting these results faster than you'd ever imagine. You see,

I challenge you to change your life and FEEL time moving backwards inside your body...

Reflexes like a *cobra,* able to respond to any attack with a raging river of *sizzling* energy.

Protected by an invisible shield where <u>strikes and punches bounce off</u> like a trampoline.

Lungs that are fully capable of resisting, and actually welcome and enjoy, the crushing forces of gravity when you crouch in low stance for extended periods of time.

So <u>everything</u> is my one-of-a-kind discovery that even I had trouble believing it's potential, but I refused to listen to mainstream propaganda about the benefits of slow motion Tai Chi for improving balance in our senior population and...blah-blah-blah. It struck me like a lightening bolt...WHY are we continuing the myth that old age needs to run in slow motion on low octane fuel...when we have the potential to regenerate our energy fuel cells and fly at light speed?

Almost every martial art out there focuses on lurking threats to your safety and well being. They promise to transform you into a fearless beast of nature. Some of them even promote different ideas on regaining vibrant health and longevity.

But even the toughest soldier of war is vulnerable to the effects of aging without discovering the core root. Which leaves you helpless as a puppy at a time of your life when tigers should use their years of experience to play and enjoy life on the dangerous thrilling edge.

The ROOT is what I'm discussing here. Hidden deep within our subconscious mind, modified from it's natural state by society so long ago that we're no longer sure of the who, what, where and why. And it's the thwarted root that causes your internal systems to break down. And that puts you on the fast track to bent over old age—*especially* when it comes to fully enjoying the martial art you spent a life time nurturing.

There's no doubt that martial arts combined with meditation has untold benefits and is probably the best way to hone life skills. Thousands of years of meditation evidence supports this. But today in the 21st century, if you want total independence to live the life originally meant for you—self-realization with heaven on earth—then you must fight against the negative influences of society. This means going deep into your core root to discover the original source of wrongful taboos implanted by society. And for most people, I believe, quiet meditation is not the most direct route to the root.

And where is the root? Locating it may not be as important as vibrating it. Your most basic instinct to survive is the surest switch to turn on the correct frequency of vibration that purifies your root. There's no doubt that instinct is your best friend here. No age-fighting program should be without instinct release in its arsenal. A pure innocent instinct will guide you through the necessary steps to freedom from disease plus invigorate you with health and vitality at any age.

If you chose meditative Tai Chi as your path to bliss but have not yet considered the role instinct plays then you may have *overlooked* DANGERS that could be putting yourself on a collision course with *old* age. This may sound like pretty heavy stuff but believe me, my discovery is an extremely simple method to help you free your boxed-up instinct. I believe I've unearthed a **golden key** that helps unleash, support and preserve your basic instinct…EVERY aspect of your health…your well being… AND your youth.

The steps that guide you to unchain your instinct are revealed in my book, *Teeth In Mortal Combat,* and in my website— *www.Tooth-Fight.com.* Incorporating them into your Tai Chi helps rejuvenate and *transform* your cardiovascular health… vision…mental clarity…digestive health…bone strength…immune system…blood sugar…muscle tone…speed…balance… stamina…and more…and most importantly, your Tai Chi is the vehicle for the process.

My book is quite literally THE SPARK YOU'VE BEEN WAITING FOR AND NEED. But unlike any other method for self-atTainment being developed and sold every day, my system works fast and true…I proved it to myself.

Teeth In Mortal Combat WILL be
your Tai Chi secret for looking and *feeling*
younger and more vibrant than
practitioners half your age!

I don't know about you, but I was told that it took 10 years of consistent Tai Chi practice to concentrate the Chi. Then another 10 years to boil it into steam. So I loaded my day with Tai Chi practice and meditation and after 20 years…nothing worth talking about…nada…and then finally, after 25 years I discovered a way to unleash my instinct to survive…and this was NOT openly taught in any class I joined.

And now I see an unbound instinct as:

An *iron-clad* foundation for
<u>ultimate longevity</u>

Which is why this book may go down in history as *the most exciting contribution to anti-aging development*. A dynamic method that could accomplish *what no other anti-aging system has ever been able to do. A hidden treasure for your youth*...

Rescue tired, worn out Tai Chi, bringing it **back from the brink of death.**
Pump NEW LIFE into your physical work out.
Increase your resistance to the diseases of society.

In other words, unleashing your basic instinct for survival using your teeth, tongue and jaws as described in the book can literally upgrade your age-fighting abilities and <u>that</u> may very well be the key to stopping aging in its tracks.

It's been an elusive secret—until now, but I'm convinced it works and it's HUGE!

And I believe it will work for YOU too!

Granted, the results are preliminary, and the research was done on myself, but this is the sort of breakthrough I've waited 25 years for. I don't want you to have to wait that long, which is why I'm sharing my discovery now.

Give your Tai Chi a fresh start --
No matter how old you are
or how many years you've be practicing.

I believe unleashing your basic instinct to survive, as described in the book, is the mother of all basic Tai Chi development. It's so unique, it's impossible to lump it together with other manuals you've read.

You see, unlike other teachings that require a Master's presence for transmission, *Teeth In Mortal Combat* touches a basic concept that is easily grasped at home after reading the details in a book. And on top of that, it may actually help revitalize other aspects of your Tai Chi training that have lost their steam after repetition and boredom. In other words, <u>the book may be the secret to getting even more benefits</u> from the practices you are already doing in shorter time (instead of adding hours of training into your daily schedule).

But what I believe really gives the book its edge is its ability to work as a life support system for ailing Tai Chi enthusiasm after years of study with no satisfactory results. It seems to re-kickstart the learning process, and then your Tai Chi can step in and carry on the work of rejuvenating your body as it is expected to. And soon you'll be on your way to

the best health of your life
with the most energy you didn't know you had
without changing a single thing in your Tai Chi!
<u>**except the way you think about your teeth.**</u>

Remember how I said that my Tai Chi didn't give decent results for close to 25 years (to put it mildly)? Well, I decided that no one should have to feel like their Tai Chi, eternal health—and YOUTH—was a burden. So I discovered the <u>simplest strategy</u> for delivering rock solid results.

And what I came up with is a remarkably easy and FUN adjustment in training that is so effective I doubt you'd complete any Tai Chi form again without inserting the principle somewhere within.

Sound too good to be true? For once, **it isn't!**

And if all this hasn't convinced you that *Teeth In Mortal Combat* is **the one support you really need in your arsenal for life, health, AND your youth,** then there's one more thing you should know...

This <u>ultimate anti-aging Tai Chi boosting solution</u> is PENNIES in price compared to what you have already paid for your martial arts study!

Normally, I hate talking about price. The way I see it, anything that improves your health—especially something as valuable as Tai Chi—is worth whatever the cost. But I'll admit it—times today are tough—people are struggling to keep their jobs and pay the mortgage on over valued houses. Every penny needs to be watched and the price of this book can save you thousands of dollars in weekend self-help and martial arts classes.

But then, again, your health and your future are well worth the investment...right?

Well, here's where this top-to-bottom, inside-out, miracle book really shines. Because it costs roughly about what you would pay for a couple of tall coffees at your local espresso cafe.

Now, it's a tiny investment. Probably the least amount of money you'll ever spend on an anti-aging, Tai Chi boosting solution. But what's packed into this extraordinary breakthrough book—the ability to rejuvenate your whole body and possibly uncoil a lifetime of negative impressions left by society, through enhanced Tai Chi—is truly an incredible value.

And unlike other programs that require you to learn... 9...12...18...36...108 and more forms and meditations than you can remember without a suitcase full of scribbled notes, you can seamlessly incorporate the main principle of the book into your day. It's almost effortless because your basic instinct to survive has dominion over all your other instincts and responds without hesitation when you give it free reign. It helps deliver powerful revitalizing effects with just a little mental effort. So you'll get *all the motivation you'll need* to build the ultimate anti-aging foundation while enhancing your practice of Tai Chi—no more boredom, no more depression, no more giving up...

All that makes this one-of-a-kind breakthrough **downright invaluable.**

Put it to the challenge and I'm convinced you'll feel *younger* and your Tai Chi will be <u>more vibrant</u> than it's been in years.

The natural basic instinct and anti-aging Tai Chi accelerating miracle that leaves other modern "gimmicks" in the dust!

But once you try it, you'll agree that it's amazing just how well this works... A completely different and affordable idea that does the job of a bagful of tricks taught at high priced classes and seminars—and <u>leaves other modern "gimmicks" in the dust</u>. Because, quite frankly, none of the modern anti-aging advancements --- the meditations, exercises, supplements, attitude adjustments—can even begin to compete with *Teeth In Mortal Combat's* astounding ability to revitalize every system and every cell in your body because it is the ONLY information that deals with your core basic instinct of survival.

Besides, you're lucky if you can remember all the details of all the classes you signed up for without the trunk of your car, where you probably store all the class handouts and notes. But give *Teeth in Mortal Combat* a try and you'll find yourself at the beginning of an incredible journey BACK IN TIME to the point where the original sperm and ovum that created you relied on survival instincts to fight incredibly hard and courageously for the honor of giving you life.

It's not just the future of Tai Chi training...it's **the future of ultimate health and longevity.** Packed into a single book of refreshingly novel and effective ideas! And inside your subconscious mind, the ideas in the book kick off an even more astounding transformation...unloading a trunk full of silly and wrongful taboos embedded by society within your subconscious mind.

So there's simply no doubt in my mind that *Teeth In Mortal Combat* is the answer to all your prayers for *living longer...feeling better... and improving your Tai Chi more* than you thought was possible. And as if the book's power to help transform and **rejuvenate** *every system in your body* wasn't enough, there's another opportunity you need to know about.

Save money for yourself and your friends while you SAVE YOUR YOUTH

Once you've experienced *Teeth In Mortal Combat's renewing,* revitalizing effects, you won't be able to bear the thought of another physical workout or Tai Chi practice without using the advice within its pages. Make sure you always have it on hand so you can share its **original primitive moving force** with your friends.

No more obscure teachings! Get every signal your body needs to neutralize aging—the original seed of survival.

Martial arts movements and meditations can pile up quick. It might start with a simple one hour class...and before you know it you're taking another weekend seminar to support your love of the art...one to focus...one to build speed...one to stretch your flexibility... Some of these formulas require repeated cycles of second and third advanced training lessons. And if you're really serious about your art, you're easily taking a class a week and an advanced seminar a month.

Now you can link ALL those lessons crammed into your memory banks and cluttering up your mental closets...with a simple, single, survival thought—*and feel great* **without leaving the comfort of your home!**

Order your exclusive copy of *Teeth In Mortal Combat*—and begin blowing away the smoke screen of deception that society has hung around your eyes.

Still having trouble "getting it?"

Tai Chi—Teeth In Mortal Combat—Longevity?
Don't see the connections?

Try:

Tai Chi—Combat,
Teeth—Longevity

Got It? Get It!

How do you get to live to a healthy 120 years—and older? Tai Chi alone isn't the answer. Folks living to a healthy 120 years—and older have discovered...

CHAPTER 35
THE HUNZA SECRET IS BETTER THAN MOST TAI CHI

The Hunza Secret!

In a small kingdom high in the Himalayas, west of Pakistan, in the valley of Hunza ...

... Men can live to be 120 years and older... experience little to no illness... and father children into their 90's.

The women of 80 look no older than 40 years old.

In the winter many of the stronger men break through thick ice-covered streams and take a swim under the ice. During the warmer months men 80, 90, and 100 years old repair old crumbling rocky roads, lifting heavy stones and boulders that would make the average American shudder with disbelief. And they work 7 days a week, 12 hours each day!

The elders enjoy competitive games of volleyball in the hot sun with men 50 years younger and, and even engage in wild violent games of polo.

Tai Chi is non-existent in this part of the world, so that isn't the reason for their health, strength and longevity. You'll be amazed to know that scientists did find the Hunza secret for longevity—

it's in their teeth!

First of all, scientific studies of the Hunza in the middle of the 20th century found that they survived harsh mountain living conditions by consuming only a little more than 1,900 calories daily with only 50 grams of protein, 36 grams of fat, and 354 grams of carbohydrates. Both protein and fat were largely of vegetable origin with about an average of 6 ounces of animal meat each day.

That's about half the protein, on-third the fat, but about the same amount of carbohydrates that the average American eats in his 3.300 calorie intake. Of course, the carbohydrate that the Hunza eat is unrefined or complex carbohydrates found in fruits, vegetable and grains, while we Americans largely eat our carbohydrates in the form of empty-nutrition white sugar and refined flour.

The Hunza were also noted for their gentle, affectionate and playful disposition. The people lived in a cooperative spirit—not competitive—and the valley of Hunza was noted as a Shangri-La of peace and contentment, free of social stress.

It makes sense that if you eat less and fewer calories, especially avoiding processed food, and live without social stress, your teeth will last your whole life. You won't suffer the consequences of bruxism—the wearing away of tooth enamel by the gnashing and grinding of teeth due to deep unresolved psychological stress—and with less food to chew the tooth enamel won't be subject to excessive natural abrasive forces. Eating and drinking an all natural diet with regular meals during the day also keeps harmful acids from attacking and dissolving tooth enamel into tooth decay. This is in stark contrast with today's American constantly snacking and sipping acidifying processed food and beverages leading to tooth decayed cavities and gum disease, modern man's most prevalent scourge of disease.

The Hunza had strong, sound, healthy teeth that lasted a lifetime and allowed them to thoroughly chew their food into a soft, mushy, enzyme rich bolus that was completely digested and utilized by their organ systems providing a happy and fruitful lifetime of rich, vibrant energy. Diamond-hard teeth are vital to good health. Completely masticated food is essential for optimal colon health with efficient digestion, absorption and utilization by the body for a long healthy life.

Ever eat corn, beans, nuts,or root vegetables—and discover whole remnants of those meals in your constipated stool?

Did you think it was because you didn't chew properly? Sure, these foods have insoluble fibers that are very difficult for your digestive tract to break down—no matter how much you chew, but these are the foods of the Hunza and their dynamic efficient teeth don't allow them to suffer constipation with visible large food remnants.

And today's leading gastroenterologists agree with me totally and unanimously when I proclaim:

It's The Teeth, DUMMY!

Take care of your teeth—and
your colon and entire body will thank you!

Longevity Is NOT The Tai Chi Form!

Longevity depends on purifying, nurturing, and harmonizing the three treasures and if you truly believe what you preach then you'll take extreme care of your teeth because it is nearly impossible to purify and nurture your body without teeth.

Yes, Tai Chi has it's many valuable benefits, but Tai Chi alone does not grant longevity. A healthy hard working lifestyle enabled with a full set of sound chompers, however, is almost certain to bless you with a long, active and satisfying life. A life where lifting boulders, dancing with younger women and fathering children at age 90 is only another day's work. And I, honestly, have not seen any of my slow, smooth-flowing, dreamy—and aged—Tai Chi friends even approaching these standards of vitality.

Enough is enough!
Your Tai Chi "stuff" doesn't work…

…If we're discussing longevity!

The way Tai Chi is being taught today is a **JOKE** among **REAL** Tai Chi Masters. And if Tai Chi suddenly arrived in Hunza-land, all elderly would be considered immediate natural Masters of child-like play. They know how to live with "fierce hoopla!"

Once you've read *Teeth In Mortal Combat,* you'll understand how your teeth play the most significant role in developing your tan-tien. Unless you've learned to breathe through your eyes, ears and skin, nothing enters the tan-tien without first passing through the nose and mouth. The teeth and jaws are critical in the first step of transmuting environmental chi into the "honey pearl drop" that you swallow into your tan-tien.

Stop putting temporary bandaids on your chi development problems. Instead, the teeth, tongue and jaws strengthen your <u>entire</u> meridian system. I've seen this work wonders in my life and it will in yours, too!

Remember when you were a teenager and could do anything? Follow the steps in my book and you'll ignite your Tai Chi fire using your teeth. You'll learn how to unleash your basic instinct for survival to turn your body system into a self-healing machine. Super-charge your sexual drive when all else failed.

Had <u>ENOUGH</u>?

<u>Enough</u> styles and weapons?

<u>Enough</u> forcing hundreds of forms into an hour of practice?

<u>Enough</u> meditations until you can barely think no-think?

BEFORE YOU ADD ANY MORE "ENOUGH"
just because "everyone" says it's necessary…

IF THE GOVERNMENT LOVES IT (as in China), IF TV PROMOTES IT, IF MOST MARTIAL ARTS SCHOOLS TEACH IT, and everyone nags you to do it, ignore it. The road to REAL TAI CHI SUCCESS isn't found in the mainstream media and it's easier, cheaper and more fun than you dared to dream!

Learn the facts of REAL TRAINING from the most unique breakthrough book that readers are calling a "myth-buster" and "taboo crusher." And let it show you how to shrug off your Tai Chi miseries in one easy step by focusing on your teeth, tongue, and jaws.

Join the martial arts world of smart readers and be DECADES AHEAD OF THE HERD!

Take most of what you read in martial arts magazines and TOSS IT IN THE TRASH!

Just say NO to the Tai Chi police…

…and feel your miseries fade away, because you are being force-fed a diet of supposedly "secret" ancient traditions that take you no-where but up a

yin-yang hole where the sun don't shine.

You rarely hear about teeth being used in exercise and combat and I believe…

**IT'S TIME TO INSPECT THE TEETH-HATERS
and find out who their contributors are.**

Some of the world's wealthiest corporations, governments, armies, and fitness "experts" are "generously supporting" one of

America's best-known body building and fitness gurus. And what is his advice?

More Government intervention in school fitness programs—**NO TEETH NEEDED!**
More buying of specialized exercise equipment—**NO TEETH NEEDED!**
More Protein Shakes—**NO TEETH NEEDED!**
More Exercise—**NO TEETH NEEDED!**
More reps—**NO TEETH NEEDED!**

Wow, how surprising.

Why Do the Authorities Keep Ignoring the Most Important Organ Group in Your Body—Teeth, Tongue and Jaw?

New evidence shows that the most life-giving organ system in your body—teeth, tongue and jaws—is totally ignored by medical, fitness and martial arts organizations. And when ignored, it causes a never-ending cycle of health problems and emotional dissatisfaction with life.

Some say "Death begins in the colon" but that is SO WRONG since NOTHING gets to the colon without first passing through the teeth and tongue. It's critical that the teeth and tongue are worked adequately and efficiently to maintain and restore the balance of good health.

The *Teeth In Mortal Combat* miracle solution makes your Tai Chi feel better and your health get better fast—as it dissolves away negative social taboos that harm our chi flow.

**"It's Like Having
32 Tiny Pearly White Doctors
Working 'Round the Clock in Your Mouth."**

And scientists are proving that MORE focus on the oral cavity is better when it comes to improving health through body and brain fitness.

"If your mouth is sick, your body is, too."

"If you want REAL RESULTS in fitness and martial arts, you need the most

Power-Packed PUNCH a healthy body can trigger.

Sick Wont Stick!

And please be advised...

If your goal is health and wealth in order to buy time for self-realization, the dreamy-sleepy Tai Chi being taught today is NOT ENOUGH to get you there. That's only because most teachers have no clue about how critical teeth are to success in life. You might be following the wrong example to guide you along the way to child-like play and personal achievement. When was the last time you saw a 90 year old Tai Chi Master dance with the step of a 25 year old or father children?

The Hunza, on the other hand, know how to dance and play with "Fierce Hoopla!" They actually live the life you're looking for and are the perfect role model for your goals. And my book is the perfect answer to strip out the mystery and secrecy behind the 3 pillars supporting superior martial arts: teeth, "fierce hoopla," and correct Tai Chi thinking.

Fierce Hoopla is the 21st Century Solution
for Drippy-Droopy Tai Chi... NOT for Dummies!

Characterized by:
Bared teeth – not clenched
Tongue pressing against the roof of the mouth

Widened eyes
Tense lower eyelids
Lowered and furrowed brows
May or may not be sinister
Difficult to interpret
Confuse your opponent

So, if you've been doing a lot of slow motion, dreamy Tai Chi and still can't play like you did when you were a child, you may not hear it but your energy system is screaming, **"SEND HELP NOW!"** It wants you to incorporate "fierce hoopla" somewhere into your Tai Chi. And my book shows you how the teeth can spark fierce hoopla into your ordinary, boring life.

Trust Your Inside.
Your Gut Knows a Good Thing When It Feels It.

Slow motion dreams have a place in your Tai Chi, but without fierce hoopla your Tai Chi is not complete. The syntropy of yin and yang will not complete and you're sure to miss the boat for longevity.

Don't sign up for another fitness class or buy another martial arts weapon until you learn more about your teeth and how to use them to unleash your basic instinct for survival through your chosen style of martial art—and my favorite is Tai Chi.

Get the Value you deserve.

Buy your copy of the book, *Teeth In Mortal Combat*...TODAY!

Chapter 36
PUT SOME WHEELS ON YOUR TRUCK

Do You Have Enough "WHEELS" On Your Truck?

THE "C.H.I.–K.I." HORMONE
and how to uncage it

C.H.I.— Commander of Human Instinct
K.I.— Knowing with Intent

**What your Sifu never
told you about how to
wipe out a lifetime of mind control**

You are about to discover the alarming reason why so many men are suffering timid dares, "sorry excuse syndrome", thinning threats, sagging defenses, dull wits, decreased performance and loss of self-confidence. And how to reverse it—FOREVER—with the most powerful instinct driven formula ever discovered.

What turns tired-out wimps into
AGELESS WINNERS?
FOUND: *The "zero point energy" of life*

Why is it? Some lucky guys live and enjoy gracefully, seemingly gaining strength and success with each passing year. You'll find these men at the top of the food-chain in virtually every walk of life. They exude power and confidence in every step. Instead of being friends with the devil of distress and failure, they're independently rugged and wise.

Younger women think they're incredibly sexy

Younger men envy them, and older men wonder...

"Why them and not me?"

Well? Why *does* Father Fate turn these fortunate few into ageless demigods...

While the rest of us slowly morph into weak, flabby, anguished old grumps who haven't taken on a decent challenge in years? I now have an answer—and I think it's going to surprise you.

It's not luck and it sure isn't clean living, following all the rules (not that there's anything wrong with either) ...

**It's a precious pearl that drips a
pure dew-like energy
flowing within every man's body.**

Yes, I'm talking about "Big ITS"—*instinct to survive*...direct from zero point energy and linked strongly with teeth and jaws. Now I realize that teeth and jaws receives almost no press other than the daily grind of preventing cavities. You would think they were some kind of unnecessary appendage to the human face... and people from West Virginia must feel this the case since West Virginia has about 40% of their population declared as toothless. And mainstream media pays no lip service to the near-miraculous role teeth play in all aspects of living. But I'm trashing that pernicious old thinking for good by revealing...

**The shocking new truth
about BIG "ITS" and TEETH**

Teeth In Mortal Combat is so important to every man's well being that I urge you to get a copy *FAST* so you can link with the success other men enjoy boosting their transformation into winners.

FACT: Winners have superior "ITS"instinct to survive. Put any two men into the same room, and the man with sharper instinct tends to dominate. Want to know who won any game? He with the best instinct wins.

FACT: Stars have superior "ITS" instinct to survive. Not just sports stars! Successful tycoons, powerful politicians and Nobel Prize winners tend to have better instinct than their counterparts who toil in dark corners, lost in obscurity.

FACT: "ITS" made you a man. The very driven, frenzied sperm that impregnated the patiently waiting egg leading to your birth had the ULTIMATE "ITS" instinct to survive. That Super Hero Sperm had to have miraculous instinct to survive, achieving a Super Olympic victory over several million other wimpy sperm. He had to bear "manly teeth" to bite through the protective cell membrane of the egg. That one mighty sperm has bragging rights to **America's Magnificent Male Authority!**

And you are so blessed to have inherited it's most distinguished gene, "ITS"... Instinct to Survive. With this gene hardwired into your energy system, you have the potential to win widespread acclaim for breakthroughs you could never imagine. World-class athletes, high-powered executives and prestigious scientists will come knocking at your door to learn your revolutionary secrets for transforming the lives of thousands.

This and MORE can be gleaned out of my most unique book. And rest assured the book has **nothing** in common with so-called expert self-help copycat books sold at bookstores or on the Internet. This is an extraordinary book not for your average "Joe" or "over the hill... it's too late... toss in the towel" loser.

And if you want to regain your manhood
You've Got To Unleash Your "ITS"

Teeth In Mortal Combat is proving to be a powerful replacement for impotent secret riddles propagated by incompetent teachers. It can slash off years of wandering through the maze of dojos claiming to hold the golden key of time tested traditions.

From now on, you don't have to settle for second best. You can NOW begin a journey to unbridled freedom to live the passion within you. Please be very careful not to waste your money on products that claim to bring results but only leave you empty handed.

You can capture the hidden secrets embedded within the fascinating lines of my book that can spark a rejuvenation of instinct you were born with and ...
Lift Yourself to Amazing New Heights.

Life has an abundance of hidden daggers that stab, slice, and then wrap up and stash away your vulnerable instincts. Without a strong guiding light you are almost defenseless against these elements, unless you feed your energy with special nutrition. This advanced and comprehensive dietary supplement is not found in a pill, powder, or liquid but it is known for its ability to help protect and rejuvenate damaged instinct while promoting the overall health of your physical, mental and spiritual being.

Scientific Research Proves ...

The dietary formula I'm speaking of is—**intention**—and when intent is used in the right way you can ...

FEEL YOUR INSTINCT SURGE
THROUGH YOUR BODY!

If you want speedy, fast improvement in your martial arts skills or just life in general, BUY the book, *Teeth In Mortal Combat*, TODAY. I was excited, surprised and couldn't imagine that a simple tinker with my daily exercise routine could deliver such powerful life transforming results in my life. After spending over 25 years searching for a results driven method, I was so happy to discover I hit pay dirt with a solution that measures up and…

I Regained My Manhood at 59!

It was so great to finally feel the satisfaction that comes with rock solid hard self-confidence. I am so grateful! And you will be too…once you make the commitment to…

…"stop taking the abuse society lays on you—right now
and TAKE BACK YOUR MANHOOD!"

Your sensitive instincts are exposed to and drowned daily in a sea of harmful negative subliminal messages controlled by big corporate fat cats, high powered government agencies and international religious and political bodies.

You have this problem right now! My research shows that your teeth and jaws are a gateway to curing you of this "Hidden Epidemic" That Sneaks Up On You…

To keep your instinct fresh and alive, I have shown that the information in my book is so powerful it helps re-ignite burned-out survival reflexes. You can count on it's valuable lessons to help you "build up" resistance to unnatural outside pressures trying to control your life. Failing instinct is NOT something that happens on your 40th, 50th, or 60th birthday…but it gradually grows sluggish over time regardless of age.

Now, do something to safeguard yourself from a "mummifying instinct for survival"—a dreadful condition that we all face living in a modern world. You will find a source of joy in protecting your future and the dreams of those you love most.

CHAPTER 37
THE GREATEST DISCOVERY

The Greatest Discovery to Enliven Your Energy
Since Shouting...Kiai!

SPECIAL REPORT: Fighting Arts Alert!

The safest way to...
Unclog Your Instincts at the
SPEED-OF-LIGHT

Your worst nightmare is now over!

Each and every word in the powerful book, *Teeth In Mortal Combat,* delivers proven results to get you on the fast track to feeling "ultimate confidence" everyday, all day...24/7. This blockbuster breakthrough—eases your fears, once and for all, about being attacked by a crazed brute.

FINALLY SOME GOOD NEWS!!. *Teeth In Mortal Combat* is the solution you need to assist you in handling any kind of imminent physical danger, extreme tournament competition, and all other bizarre, aggressive behavior stacking overwhelming odds against you.

Guaranteed to loosen handcuffed instincts
that can up-shift your self-defense skills
beyond your imagination!

Transform your Fighting Style using instincts
once frozen by societal taboos and feel stronger,
energized, and more confident

than you ever thought possible...
...RIGHT NOW!

YOUR FUTURE BEGINS NOW!
Make the Rest of Your Life, the Best of Your Life!

Teeth In Mortal Combat Outperforms
All Competitors On The Market!
It Works—And It Works Fast!

Smacked and dropped to your knees, having your purse stolen, being assaulted in the city, getting car-jacked—these are among the life-threatening consequences of big city life, the Number One Cause of Stress... it's the Modern Living Silent Epidemic.

If you—or anyone you love—has ever had
a life-threatening experience...
This is The Most Important Report you will ever read!

Dear Lover of the Fighting Arts,

I know firsthand that danger lurks at every corner and there usually aren't any warning signs. if your instincts aren't sharp as a razor, your life could be at risk.

When I was struggling through school, working a night time job, I was grabbed at gun point, pushed into the back seat of a car, and driven away to be robbed and then ditched in some unfamiliar woods. That's when I dedicated myself to finding effective approaches to preventing bodily harm from the growing epidemic of crime facing the United States. I can't relive my frightful school day experience in order to change the memories. But, perhaps, I can help you avoid the agonizing paranoia that follows similar frightening hostile encounters.

Here are the shocking facts: By the time you finish reading this report, if you live in a big city, a dozen people within a 3 mile radius of you will have been threatened with bodily harm in some sinister way. Just living in this stressful environment can affect your health and well being. Will you or a member of your family be the next to fall victim to some unpredictable, demented, abhorrent event so common in America... Tomorrow's News Headlines?

Revitalize Your Self-Defense Instincts
and Natural Ability to Survive Danger
At An Astonishing Speed With
The Most Powerful, Common Sense Solutions
Ever Found In One Book... Now Available To You

A blanket of protection 24 hours a day, 7 days a week,
365 days a year... what more can you wish for?!

There Are No Substitutions for Keen Instincts

That's why I searched every corner of alternative and traditional teachings to help find the best way to spark instinct alive again, in a growing epidemic of societal choke-holding taboos.

Thanks to my exhaustive search, I believe a secret has finally been uncovered to help unleash superior **instincts at any age.** *Teeth In Mortal Combat* is a book that ignites the battle against a society that constantly invents ways to crush our instincts... but now you can **break free** and benefit whether you are 18, 30, 50, 90... or even older than 100 years old.

I believe my book is the best measure to fully unlock and develop your basic instinct for survival before any further serious problems creep up in your life. Remember the old saying..."An ounce of prevention is better than a pound of cure."

Your Efforts Will Pay Off!

I've proven... That It Works...
And It Works Unbelievably Fast!!

It is my sincere desire and personal goal to help you take the unnecessary worry out of life and make you feel happy again! My book will definitely be able to give you the initial support to you or anyone you love who may suffering under the unbearable heaviness of society's system of repression. Everyone now has access to a revolutionary new way to keep their genetic instincts feeling young and vibrant.

This **Amazing Breakthrough Book** and its **great unrestrained power** can help resolve your confusion about what it is that is keeping you from succeeding. After reading it, you can truly begin "peeling off the forbidden layers of your onion" and, like a dog coming out of water after a swim, shake yourself free of all the mind controlling games society secretly plays.

This Book Is Paying Off in the Fight for Success,
Health, Safety, and Peace

I know all too well what it is like losing control of your life to adversaries, including the overbearing artificial rules of society. My goal is that every person has the means to unravel the sham, restrictive rules of society fettering access to our most basic life instincts. My book will help open your eyes to the potential miraculous relief you can experience for the first time in years.

Teeth In Mortal Combat, with the very First Page, Will Begin Blasting Away Manipulating Taboos and...
... Put YOU Back in the Saddle!

My book is the "Anti-Control" solution for instinct that stopped feeding your energy directly to your reflexes. If over the years you've had too much mental conditioning overriding free reign of your basic instincts, you become a major candidate for political manipulation. We know that the most powerful institutions on earth carefully select psycho-suggestive formulas to maintain control of the populace. But the condition is not hopeless, which is why I uncover little know theories about the intellectual and spiritual castration of the human race.

Usually, taboos instigated by malevolent rulers start being enforced at an early age. Since ancient time these subjugating taboos became so much a part of normal life that no one feels the need to question them. The harm they cause, however, can tattoo small chinks in our armor which then rusts up. If these rusty chinks reach a certain size, they can cause you to freeze up during competition, slow down your reflexes, make you a walking target for crime and, in general, clog up your energy system so that your once bubbling instinct is unable to function when you need it most.

Teeth In Mortal Combat
Can Revitalize Your
Basic Instinct For Survival...

...making for fast positive progress because your intention starts the river of energy flowing to your heart fast...giving you an energy boost that doesn't quit...when and where you need it most.

Right now you could be breaking out of inconvenient handcuffs, put in place by society, that keep your infinite energetic potential from becoming all that you can be. Read my book and immunize yourself against dangerous negative viral influences trying to take over your health and wealth by *stealth*. Statistics show it's now getting worse year by year. It affects people of all ages…women and men…young adults and teens and, frightening enough, even innocent infants and children. No one seems to be immune to this potentially life-threatening threat. Now there is still time for you to **fight this tragedy with my** *dynamic* **book before it's too late.**

The Ideas in Teeth In Mortal Combat Go Instantly Into Your Life Force Where It Is Needed Most

Zero Point Energy for Your Genetic Code that Reminds Your DNA How, What, Where, and When to Fully Express Itself…
Unlimited Instinct with NO Think…to Get It Done!

CHAPTER 38
THE SHARPER INSTINCT
REVOLUTION

The Sharper Instinct Revolution

Critical Report For Those with Shaky, Anemic,
Undependable Instinct

Your Instinct is the Passport to the World

With This Astonishing Breakthrough by a Dentist
You Can Help Unleash Your Instinct Gummed up from
Years of Living Under Big Brother's Heavy Hand

Can You Think of Anything More
Devastating Than Living with Wobbly Instinct?

Sharp Instinct Come From
Sharp Awareness

"Unleash your instinct" means to be totally aware both day
and night, 24/7. Your instinct is your most important tool for
survival and it needs to be protected. The discoveries revealed in
Teeth In Mortal Combat may be your best defense against the terrible affects society's power hungry forces have on your instinct.
You now have the opportunity to experience the unrivaled brawn
of self-determination…the sensational formula for dominion
over your life is in your hands…and you can have strong unfet-
tered instinct for the rest of your life—AGELESS FREEDOM!

Are YOU ready to beat
THE "SHAKY INSTINCT" BULLET?

This astonishing new secret technique may be the
extra horsepower that delivers brilliant, ultra-clear, and
maximum rejuvenation to your instinct for survival.

React with confidence, banish negative thought…
look and move as one capable dynamic fury.
And you, too, can belong to the special group of warriors
whose instinct gets better day by day.
Your life will never be the same!

In Only Days, You Can Have Sharper and Clearer Instinct!
—And Protect Yourself From The Crippling Pressure of
Unnatural Taboos Forced On You By Society!
It Really Works With Unbelievable Results!

Having studied theories from some of the most
brilliant minds in the martial arts,
I can honestly say that this is one of the most effective ways
to get in touch with your instinct today!
I believe it has no equal and am very proud of it.

Dear Freedom Loving Friend,

Have you ever wished you had a "freedom" doctor in your
family? Someone you could trust to give you dependable advice
about caring for your instinct to survive and be free? This dramatic new breakthrough book, for cleansing and improving spotty
instinct, can help promote your overall precious right to not only
survive in today's turbulent times but also thrive with your personal vision of an unlimited future.

If you add just one tiny tool to your current workout and
meditation routine, it definitely should be for your instinct to

survive. Your survival instinct training is your most important and precious friend, completely different from other parts of your exercise sets. Responsive instinct depends on many factors. Healthy robust cell vigor and energy flow, as well as an awareness of the reality of life. Your instinct should be fed with wisdom, the manna of the ancient sages.

Teeth In Mortal Combat uncloaks a powerful snapshot of what's really happening in your life, preventing you from nourishing your instinct for survival and keeping it as strong as it should be. In addition, it has techniques that help unclog sluggish mental and physical reactions to danger. They encourage regular support to fight back against repressive local and world powers.

Most people don't think much about the impairment of their correct response to everyday situations. What begins as merely an inconvenience can with time grow into a debilitating and deteriorating robbery of our independence, stealing life's greatest pleasures.

Imagine what your life would be like if you were totally dependent on others to make decisions for you in your daily activities you now take for granted. This is exactly what is happening to us, to some degree. Some futurists even believe that some day the average person will ultimately LOSE INDEPENDENCE.

Don't let this serious
problem happen to you!

Only in recent years have researchers started figuring out the secrets hidden in ancient Chinese and Hindu texts that connect the energy meridians running through the major organs and teeth with health and emotional disposition…and all their hard work is paying off for you, for me and for everyone who wants—and needs—to free up rusting instincts—so we can hold on to the independence to react to life's daily challenges in the way that is best for each of us.

The hidden secret to sharp instinct, clear confident reaction, and proper interpretation of life's signals is directly linked with your teeth and jaws.

For many years I searched and studied top teachers with strong knowledge in instinct—people who could make you feel and perform more efficiently... help rejuvenate and bring instinct to a higher level. These teachers were on a mission: To find the best way that could easily help thousands to develop their energy in spite of modern day disruptions.

In younger years, your energy flows relatively unobstructed and able to react naturally. As you get older, taboos enforced by society clog the circulation of energy and by the time you reach 35–40 years old, layers of taboos slowly block your instinct from guiding you and, if nothing is done, can over the years lock you in a prison of self-doubt. That is why it is so essential to start breaking the prison chains link by link as soon as you become aware of your "disability."

The information uncovered in my book helps blast away unhealthy energy blocks. You can now effectively wash your meridians clean. Senseless taboos begin to dissolve in your mind leading to the opening of a free flow of energy throughout your body—eliminating any uncertainties from your life.

This extraordinary development in training can help stimulate the flow of energy, through intention, to support your entire fabric for survival. You can feel like you did when you were 10, 20, or 30 years younger. Even better, you can wipe out a lifetime of fear based decisions and regain your manhood!

306   Teeth In Mortal Combat — *Bonus Chapters*

What does this mean for you? It means now, instead of being a helpless victim of society's choking squeeze, you can reverse the layers of negativity and become a triumphant victor over life's challenges.

Revealed for the first time…
Secrets to Better Unobstructed Instinct

The synergistic array of scientific facts and theories found in *Teeth In Mortal Combat* offers a unique perspective on uncovering your emotional response to using teeth and jaws in battle, to help slow down and even reverse the further deterioration of your instinct for survival. You shouldn't be without this remarkable book which is so important for unrestrained instinct—for strengthening and providing clearer action and response to your infinite visions.

Before this book was written, there wasn't very much that you could do at home, without personal and costly instruction from a qualified teacher, to unravel the mysterious connection between your teeth, jaws, and instinct for survival. Now, that's all changed! Just think, you may never have to worry again about the right way and wrong way. Read the book, change your daily practice in tiny simple ways, and never worry again when you go with your gut feelings.

Teeth In Mortal Combat dramatically opens your eyes to the harmful effects of society's controlling taboos, especially when associated with teeth and jaws. You'll learn what your teacher never told you: *how to unleash your most basic instinct for survival.*

CHAPTER 39
THE SILENT ASSASSIN

This *Silent Assassin*
Triples Your Risk of Getting Clobbered
Physically and Mentally

*... but most martial artists are at risk and don't even know it.
How to tell if you are and what you can do about it.*

As someone who cares about your body and mind, you try to avoid contaminated food, drink, air, and negative thoughts. You try to exercise and learn self-defense skills.

But despite your healthy intentions, you may still be at risk for a gut-wrenching, head banging, freedom stealing, mind control conspiracy. You see, there is a silent assassin stalking you.

This silent assassin hypnotizes you and overtakes your free will; mesmerizes your basic instinct for survival. And you never see it coming, not even knowing you were at risk.

So what is this silent assassin? It's the disease of "SCREAMING SCREEN!"

Screaming Screen disease has three main routes of attack:

Television Screen

Movie Screen

Computer Screen

Now I know what you're thinking. "I'm not at risk for the the SCREAMING SCREEN." I hope that's true. I hope you're making lifestyle choices that will lower your chances.

Maybe you're watching educational documentaries, enjoying films that feature uplifting positive messages with healthy core values, studying online to get a college degree, searching for new meditation techniques. They are all very effective for self-improvement.

But a healthy lifestyle filled with pure uplifting entertainment and education may still not be enough to protect you from the Screaming Screen. We all have one risk factor for developing this disease. It's a hidden cause.

So what is the hidden cause?

It's Low Energy!

Now I'm not talking about feeling tired and rundown. It seems that nearly everyone that lives a typical modern lifestyle feels that way these days.

When I say "low energy," I'm talking about low energy in your brain cells and in the spirit of your instincts. Having poor energy production not only puts you at risk of the Screaming Screen. Poor energy production also leads to many other serious problems such as making poor choices in life, not having enough money, falling into unworkable relationships, not smelling the dirt in the dump, not seeing the truth from the hype.

As you know, our natural born instinct is the truest arrow pointing us toward self-realization, success, and happiness. And our brain cells are the physical dimension connecting and controlling our life energy with the free flow of instinct. And when these brain cells work efficiently, your energy production—physical, mental, and spiritual—burn a path for you to greater freedom of expression.

The problem with the Screaming Screen is that it can affect your entire being at all levels, in negative ways, by turning down your energy producing functions. And when your energy production drops, your brain pathways start to short circuit, strapping tight your free flow of life dependent instincts.

Today, our culture of the Internet is doing something no one could have predicted. It's a curious psychological phenomenon which allows people to react virtually with online chats where you can vent and rant, releasing pent up energy while never actually stepping out the door to do something about the truth of our evaporating freedoms. The trend may become more serious in the years ahead as television, movie, and computer screens induce us into a passivity never before seen.

It would be well to review the actual meanings behind the word "screen." While a screen can actually protect when used thoughtfully, it also has many negative meanings which can subvert our consciousness:

1.) A movable device designed to divide, and conceal.
2.) Something that divides.
3.) A block that impedes vision or movement.

Now you can start to see the negative cycle that starts to develop from sitting behind a screen for too many consecutive hours. First, brain cells become overwhelmed with too much information. Then they short circuit and fail to signal energy production from within the body's energy producing cells. The brain, heart, and mind act on an intimate level of cooperation and their complex workings will eventually erode into poor decision making, crippling the instinct for survival.

How to Cure the Illness by Fixing the Root Cause

I'm not suggesting that you avoid the "Screen" or develop a fear of it. The good news is that when you are aware of the problem, you can not only control it, but eliminate it altogether! That's because trying to live a healthy productive life isn't enough. You have to get down right to the root of the problem, which is giving up control to the screen.

And you can find out how to stop giving up control in my ground-breaking book, *Teeth In Mortal Combat*. Some of the answers are also on this website in the article: **Anything is Possible on a Farm.**

If you're already suffering from the Screaming Screen, I'll tell you exactly how you can reverse this terrible disease inside my book and this website. Even if you don't have the Screaming Screen, the life-changing information I share in this book will help you feel younger, have more energy, and avoid ever suffering from the debilitating effects of the fast growing epidemic of locked up energy and instinct.

There is more good news. If you know what signs to look for—you can start making changes today—you can stop the Screaming Screen from happening to you.

Steps That Can Save Your Life

In my breakthrough book I not only explain exactly how giving up control leads to rusty instincts, I outline steps you can take to eliminate your chances of suffering a life where your basic instinct for survival is locked up in a steel cage. Most of my recommendations are shockingly easy to follow. Best yet, they'll all result in you feeling healthier, having more energy almost immediately, and knowing you are behind the wheels of your truck with all gears shifting.

The recommendations you'll find in this life-changing book won't just help you or someone you love avoid the Screaming Screen.

Inside its pages, you'll discover secrets that will give you back the energy and follow-your-gut instincts you used to feel many years ago.

So...if you want...

Information You Won't Find *Anywhere* Else
That Delivers Results Which Will Have You
Bursting with Energy...Glowing with Vitality, Health
and a Confident Feeling of Self-Determination...

Buy The Book NOW!

CHAPTER 40
VIVA LAS OVUM!

Ladies
Proof Just In…
YOU WIN!

Teeth In Mortal Combat might sound like a book geared to the He-Manly Hormone Fraternity, but that's far from the truth. The book reveals how to unleash your instinct to survive, a "forgotten" emotional vitamin critical to both a guy's and lady's well being.

WHY? Just look at the world around you and dissect all the taboos society restrains you with, like a giant body wrap twisting tighter and tighter around your freedom of expression and direction…a long list of no-nos…and the great majority of them are directed at women:

> No, don't do that…
> No, don't wear this…
> No, do it this way…
> No, just put up with it…
> No, you can't…
> No, you're supposed to…
> And where do all the No's take you?

No Where But
Low Self-Esteem—Depression—Failure!

Ladies, your world is brimming with taboos that make it impossible to balance all your responsibilities while allowing you to live the life of your dreams. Ouch! And you don't need another prescription drug to help you cope. What you DO need are effective strategies that unclog your sluggish instinct to help you make the right decisions that come straight from your deepest inner being. And Science is proving that women beat men, hands down, when it comes to making the best choices for the survival of our species.

It only took the male dominated scientific world thousands of years to come to the recent conclusion and truth:

Women control the very important process of safely guiding the birth and development of the species through complex internal chemical structure and tricks. We now know that the egg can select or eject the sperm of its choice.

We also know about parthenogenesis, a biologic process where the female's eggs start dividing without being fertilized. It was first observed in sharks and is one of the reasons switching from sexual reproduction to virgin birth has helped these creatures to exist on earth several hundred million years. And it is generally accepted by enlightened scientists that, to safeguard the propagation of the human race, virgin birth is possible with women by some simple switches in their biochemical mechanisms.

And this takes instinct to levels we never dreamed. Which is why women today, more than ever, need to keep their instincts fresh and free from the negative influence of mainstream media and its power driven moguls.

The problem is an overbearing society (definitely not in your best interest) limiting your choices by immersing you into its thickened soup "plot"—sorry, I meant "pot"—of world domination. A process since birth, so slow it's almost undetectable without taking a long pause to see what you have, how you got it, and most important—Do You Want It?

**Imagine scrubbing society's negative influence away
with a book like *Teeth In Mortal Combat!***

Astonishing! Ridiculous?
Try Proving It Wrong!

I believe the book is just short of a miracle for uncovering the truth and giving effective solutions to resolve abnormal rhythms in your instinct response. It's an almost instant cure for ridiculous taboos sewn into the fabric of your life and many times more effective than what self-help gurus dish out on cable networks and social media blogs.

The discoveries in the book are so shocking, you may think I'm kidding. Teeth, tongue and jaw explain away centuries of homocentric views cracking the egg as a powerful symbol of fertility? Biting and grinding issues related with the archaic ideology that women are a mere vessel for the embryo to develop? Hieronymus Fabricius. aka "the father of embryology" proclaiming that "semen perfects the egg"?

The book has answers to the origins of these male-centered views—if you are READY to accept them and TRY for 30 days the antidote prescription written especially with YOU in mind.

Now, are you ready for this?

The theories in the book are so compelling that corporate giants are desperately downplaying any remotely possible buddy-buddy partnerships they secretly hushed-up and covered-up in their quest for your soul. And the end result of their tinkering with your decision making abilities is a watering down of your capability to use your instinct for survival. In a few gritty words— they put a leash on you and are taking you for a walk.

Women and Men Alike...
you CAN put a STOP to this by becoming aware of
The Dangerous Truth About How Your Instinct
Has Been Highjacked!

LIVE AGAIN, TOTALLY FREE!

You never would have guessed it, but the teeth, tongue and jaws are critical components of the energetic continuum where instinct flows freely. And if you're agonizing for relief from dead-end life situations... and if you wonder if the answers in the book will work for you... See For Yourself!

Give it your best once over... and I guarantee you'll be satisfied and get delivered everything you expected.

Buy The Book, NOW!

Chapter 41
50 REASONS TO ACT NOW...
WITH ONE "STRONG" WARNING!

- Learn Teeth Sense with the Teeth Sensei
- In the beginning, self-defense relied on the most basic weapon—Sharp Teeth and Strong Jaws.
- Teeth and Jaws need to be strengthened in the *Spirit of the Warrior.*
- ...have a greater understanding of what it means to truly live FREE as a human being. Freedom to express your most *Basic Instinct for Survival.*
- Soon thousands of smart minded martial artists will flock to teachers that develop teeth, tongue, and jaws.
- Quite frankly, mainstream martial arts is stumped when it comes to the teeth and jaws. They don't understand why they're important, how they work, or how to develop them.
- Discover why teachers keep ignoring the most important weapon in your body.
- Teeth and Jaw Fitness should be <u>Alongside All Fitness Protocols</u>. If you are serious about your martial arts, you should consider focusing some of your ENERGY on the teeth, tongue and jaws...
- Don't make this mistake: Thinking healthy exercise and breathing techniques are all you need. People like you tell me this all the time: *They don't need another exercise to practice!* Well I'm here to tell you that if you don't have strong *HEALTHY* teeth, tongue and jaws, your meridians can't flow efficiently and you'll have a tough time containing chi—*period.* That's

why every Master I know started his training as a young child or man when the teeth and jaws are in peak health.

- Teeth training may also affect brain fitness ... increasing blood flow to the brain.
- Keep your memory, wits, and independence as this book may actually refresh your instincts.
- The study of tooth, tongue, and jaw... is the revelation of birth, life, and death.
- The teeth and tongue are gatekeepers of your body, heart and soul. NOTHING enters the inner realm of your castle without their permission. They separate useful from foul. They attack inedible demons trying to terrorize your life force and then spit the negative energy out. Grateful and loving, they honor Mother Earth's food for life, transforming molecular manna into beneficial healing energies.
- You have a birthright to express your instincts!
- It is estimated that 90% of humans have the same major energy meridian BLOCKED.
- ...if a martial artist pays special attention to and develops the chi of teeth and jaws, his/her overall fighting skills will improve.
- Isn't it about time you turn the tables in YOUR favor? Discover the one little secret for REAL LIFE results...
- **Stop mind control in its tracks!** This book has a solution for overbearing governments and controlling organizations, so simple and effective it's positively revolutionary.
- It's proving to be a huge help for correcting minor bite problems... some say it stopped jaw popping... in some cases TMD pain was relieved (temporal mandibular joint discomfort).
- It is easier for a camel to enter and walk through the eye tooth of a martial artist than it is for a Master to give you the keys to his skill.

- If you come to a master for training and he busts your chops, are you going to cry and ask for your money back?
- When you incorporate teeth into your training... follow these 5 rules...
- What you have just read is suckling milk to whet your appetite. If you really want the meat, you need a Master to prechew your meal and then transfer it to you. Without the Master's extraordinary enzymes, nature's banquet might be hard to digest.
- Something you should know... Anything is Possible on a Farm!
- Do YOU need PranaChiKiManna Hoopla Juice?
- The Joy of Dancing with Hoopla! and Ferocity!
- After reading this book, you'll have the *'juice and punch'* to feel like you never imagined possible.
- Teeth, tongue, and jaw training increases salivary flow which releases a surge of insulin. The insulin leads to an increased heart rate and sends glucose and oxygen to our brain.
- The result? This blast of brain food helps us learn faster and retain information longer.
- Attack and conquer with your... *teeth?*... Strange but true.
- "Why didn't my teacher tell me about this?" *Great question.* I know this much... it's not his fault. Incredibly, the teeth, tongue and jaws are hardly even mentioned in the ancient texts. And martial arts teachers are often threatened by societal taboos. That's why thousands of practitioners are flocking to buy my book.
- *Teeth in Mortal Combat* pushes beyond the martial artist's "comfort zone." Challenging stale assumptions. Coming up with a dazzling new solution to a puzzle that eluded tradition-bound practitioners for centuries.

- ...TURNING MEN INTO WARRIORS.
- Thankfully, your most basic instinct for survival no longer needs to be held chained and cuffed by big government or societal powers that crave more control.
- The warrior is supreme and must not do what feels good now, but should figure out what is in his/her long-term best self-interest. He/she should not give in to sudden fancies, but persevere in long-term beneficial goals. *"I count him braver who overcomes his desires than him who conquers his enemies, for the hardest victory is over self."* —Aristotle
- The discoveries revealed in this book are so POWERFUL they could be considered a *"threat"* to all governments, cults, and most of society's organized institutions.
- Every martial artist that feels a little *'behind the curve'* should know the truth about teeth in mortal combat.
- **WARNING!**: Do not train teeth and jaws before reading detailed instructions and getting a thorough dental and medical exam!
- It's true. The material discussed in this book is so "dangerous", its a MIRACLE I chanced upon it.
- ...yet if done safely, after a thorough dental exam by your dentist, it can be a truly miraculous confidence builder and skill enhancer.
- It's time to end the coverup. Despite what society would have you believe, teeth in mortal combat may save your life.
- More research is needed, but this could prove to be the biggest self-confidence breakthrough of our time.
- Start feeling the difference in months, days... or *minutes.*
- After 150 years of trying, dentists still can't cure TMJ pain. That's why I'm really rocking the boat suggesting that the

information revealed in my book, in addition to nutrition, exercise, and meditation, might do just that—reverse TMJ pain.

- Could the secret to saving your life be found in a ... SMILE?
- Unlock your body's secret fighters—**Isn't it time you learned about them right now?**
- In fact, the best way to defeat your opponent is already inside you waiting to work wonders, you just need to know how to use it...
- Whether you want to restore your own 'fight', or help a parent, spouse, or loved one... *Teeth in Mortal Combat* will show you how to get more zest out of your workout than you ever dreamed, without spending hundreds or thousands of dollars on gimmicky wacky workout videos, exercise machines, and health club contracts.
- *Teeth in Mortal Combat* study will increase your ability to concentrate.
- Feel Healthy, Look Sprightly, Be Stronger, Live Longer... with a Fierce Smile!
- The proof on this revealed secret is going to knock the dojo 'nuts' right out of their black belts!
- Step into your amazing new world where miracles can happen... Make them happen today!

Buy the Book NOW!

CHAPTER 42
MOLAR COMBAT WITH LAUGHING BUDDHA

Molar Combat
with
Killer White Teeth
and
Massive Jaws

Discover Survival Instincts Behind the
Secret Smile of Laughing Buddha

Lifting the Curtain of Mystery is a ritual practiced by all wanna-be martial artists. You have chosen this moment in time to be here with me; to catch a glimpse behind the curtain. I honor you for that and will share some of my very personal experiences with you.

I have discovered treasures in the practice of martial arts. Perfection as a goal can paralyze movement. The path is a journey of error. Questions chisel away fear; fearless, one respects power. To be a Master, detach from your Master.

In my opinion, the blinding snowy mountains of martial art styles do not have a unifying original source, as some may claim. There is no one rooted tree of self-defense from which all the others branched out. We find no movement that is simple, pure, undiluted, and therefore, more powerful and effective than all the others.

Think of a wintry blue sky thick with humid snow clouds that condense and crystallize the first original snowflakes. Which snowflake hits the solid earth first to hold the distinction of being the authentic one? Is that the snowflake we should try to recreate and imitate in our martial art fighting style? Is that the form that holds the superior wisdom, strength, and effectiveness we are searching for?

Clouds do not compete for the title "Creator of First Snowflake." Snow flakes don't fall from the sky racing to be the first landing on earth. I believe we waste precious time arguing one fighting style superiority over another. There is no single original martial art more effective and deadly than the others after it. There is no one movement that defeats all others.

It is impossible to imagine the very first snowflake that gently touched earth's highest mountain peak. Were humans there to discover, preserve, and label it? Who today can claim and prove direct lineage to this venerable form?

Yes, most researchers agree that no two snowflakes are alike. No two crystals grow into exact twins. The snow crystals, as they float and dance in flight downward to solid ground do, however, travel together. They all grow in synchrony, each having a unique and intricate design with recognizable symmetry. The same logic can be applied to the various martial arts.

What peaks my curiosity is that something appears to exists behind common symmetry. For lack of a better word, I call it "instinct". Humans today still turn to instinct for survival. It is the basis for all self-defense.

In this book I reveal an instinct common to all, from infant to adult. It is this distinct instinct that sparks all the necessary forces needed to recreate human life. Beginning at birth it feeds, protects, and preserves human life form until the day we decide to pass from this earth.

From my own experience, I believe society can depress, deform, corrupt, and mutate an individual's elemental expression of instinct. Instinct breathes life into the symmetry that exists in all of us, yet dwells suppressed, crippled, or dormant in most of us. In this book I try to define, explain, and release our birthright to an instinct nearly buried among society's artificial concepts, rules, and misconceptions. I hope that after reading this book you will have a greater understanding of what it means to truly live free as a human being. Freedom to express our most basic instinct for survival.

These and more pearls are revealed in this book. They are found hidden behind The Secret Smile of Laughing Buddha. It is my sincere wish that you benefit from this book. As a "tickler," you will learn why I believe "Molar Combat with Killer White Teeth and Massive Jaws" is one of the secrets to immortality.

I sincerely hope that the turbulent joys and sorrows of my 25 years studying the mysteries of the East will benefit you ten fold.

Sincerely, with no holds barred,
Lester Sawicki, DDS

Chapter 43
ANYTHING CAN HAPPEN ON A FARM

Dear City Born Friend,

Welcome to the Tooth-Fight/TeethSensei website where I hope you will benefit immensely from the wide spectrum of information and opinions shared.

First, allow me to explain my use of the word "sensei" as it may be a source of unintended misunderstanding. The term "sensei" refers in Japanese to persons of respect and/or leadership. These include school teachers, teachers of martial arts, doctors, politicians and some other kinds of people. In modern times this is just a polite addressing, while in the traditional way (martial arts etc.) the term includes the concept of "spiritual leader."

I use the word as a polite addressing for a dentist with experience in good "teeth sense" and "teethsensei" became a natural extension. I am not a Master of the martial arts although I have studied and practice tai chi, hard and soft qi gong, and various health and fitness exercises, plus meditation. I have met many and studied with several Masters and am very certain, in my mind, how to define one.

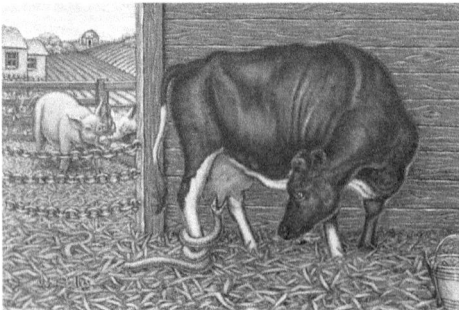

The artwork in this website might surprise and even shock you. My apologies if they offend your sense of propriety, but it is my responsibility to gain your attention and help raise your awareness through visual tools. I commissioned the art in this website and there is meaning and purpose for all the pictures. The main theme is the "Farm" and there are true stories behind the cow, snake, pig, and foal pictorials. The actual events have been transmitted through several generations of my Eastern European Polish farming family (on my father's side) and are treasured as a source of understanding and inspiration based on the saying: "anything is possible on a farm."

A young foal had tangled its head in the fence adjoining a pig pen. A hungry mature pig instinctively saw an opportunity to feed itself a "happy meal." Unfortunately, late to the rescue, my grandfather had to put down the foal.

Early one morning my grandmother discovered a snake climbing the leg of a milking cow marked with evidence of spilt milk. Most say that a milk snake is not capable of suckling milk and is a myth among farmers. There may be truth to that, but my grandmother begged to differ.

Instinct rules on a farm and is integral to the origin and continuation of life. Instinct guides us through wild adventure, peril, and insecurity. Life in itself is insecure and if you want a richer existence you must be ready to move into the unknown where the ultimate is achieved through both effort and understanding.

The wise farmer expects discomfort but never lives in misery. All his efforts gather energy to prepare the plantings and animals for death and he makes good use of death to create new life. He is not concerned with perfection and worships the flow of wholeness. Walking slowly amongst his plants and animals his awareness becomes as "one," where language is meaningless. He doesn't search what to do, but rather, how to be.

Unfortunately, our family farm was decimated during World War II. My grandparents and parents, along with most of my aunts, uncles, cousins, and their close friends emigrated to the United States of America in search of a new beginning with rumored endless opportunities. I was the first generation born in the U.S.A. and, unlike my father when he was a young farm boy, never walked the earth without shoes. The only farm I was familiar with was shown on television as Lassie's home. I have never milked a cow, fed pigs, nor raised a foal.

Most significant is that from the stories my family related, all my relations born and raised on a farm were healthy and strong, without tooth decay or gum disease, until they adopted an American lifestyle which appeared to lead them down the path of weakness and disease. They developed the typical modern Western conditions of heart disease, diabetes, and cancer...all relatively rare on the farms in their small home town.

*****

Anything Can Happen on a Farm — Part II

I have been studying exercise, nutrition, and meditation for 26 years in order to find the best ways to support and maintain excellent health in a rich, meaningful, and happy life. What I have discovered is that, contrary to the popular belief in a potential anti-aging pill that you can put in the palm of your hand, fitness and health come with constant attention to the goal. I finally connected the dots and realized that all my puzzling and very complex questions were answered simply by returning to the roots of my family's farming ancestry — peak survival by constant attention to nurturing life on the farm with a sunrise to sunset work ethic.

My challenge was to adopt a country lifestyle and find a way to implement it while living in the big city — no easy task!

After many hours of mental sweat, I wiped my brow dry and realized...

I HAD TO QUIT
BIG CITY LIFE *FOR GOOD!*

...but I didn't have to leave the city for the country!

When I compared the average typical American lifestyle with historical life on a farm, surprisingly many similarities became evident. The one major difference was how mindful attention was focused for nurturing life. The farmer of former times had fewer choices to make and less distraction from his instinctive desire to understand the wholeness of life. Current scientific studies suggest that modern America has too many choices and is unnaturally focused on the minute details of choosing one label over another, both of which lead to a lack of happiness and fulfillment.

I'm going to bluntly state that I'm not the world's smartest guy, but when I tripped over what I believe to be true underground secrets that deliver results where modern "theories" fail... I shouted...

"I'm not going to take it anymore!"

...I've had enough, trashed my current big city daily routine, broke free from the money-hungry ridiculousness of modern living and started to *really live* life for REAL again.

Look what happened over the next 45 days...
More Energy
Tighter Muscle Tone
Greater Enthusiasm
Spontaneous Exhilarating Laughter

Near 2 Inches OFF my waistline
A Greater Sense of Time and Place
Wider Smiles
Sharper Focus
Awareness Sky Rockets

It's not just another fad. In 6 weeks, it truly changed my life!

Life just got easier... and healthier... and with better fitness and fun ... and I believe you too can escape your fate ... by making one little change in your daily routine ... and the next time you see your medical doctor he'll say "Wow! I Can't Believe it!"

What I'm about to give you is the BEST News Your Doctor and Fitness Trainer Never told you ... **Improved blood oxygenation in every corner of your body.**

*****

Anything Can Happen on a Farm — Part III

Most people think we peak physically sometime in our 30's and begin to go downhill as we age with aches, pains, stiff limbs, and decreased organ function. Eventually illness and diseases like diabetes, osteoporosis, or heart disease set in. Your body begins to grow frail, weak, and basically starts to fall apart. Finally, you spend your last years in a nursing home.

This doesn't have to happen to you! Don't believe that the downward cycle of physical and mental energy is natural and inevitable. The truth is: you don't suffer a loss of energy because you age; a drop off in cellular energy causes you to age.

Every cell needs energy to function and the less energy your cells have, the poorer your body functions. If your cells aren't producing energy as effectively as they should be, you'll fall into the trap of illness and disease.

If you want to slow down, and even reverse, aging. If you want to prevent and also cure disease, then all you have to do is get your cells to increase their energy level output. The most basic solution to this is to increase the efficiency of lung function and oxygen utilization. Flood your cells with oxygen, the oxygen enters the mitochondria, energy is produced, and the resulting waste product, carbon dioxide, is expelled through the lungs.

Lung function is one of the most accurate bio-energy markers of health. The cheapest, easiest, and most practical way to increase lung function and oxygen utilization is through exercise. When it comes to exercise, however, most people either exercise too hard or they don't exercise enough.

If you don't exercise enough, your energy production furnace of mitochondria won't completely turn on and you could feel sluggish and tired. If you exercise too much, you might feel energized but you are going to create too much oxidative stress with highly reactive free radicals that can damage cells, making your body age even faster.

There are few exercise programs that test and measure lung function on a regular routine basis, but there are some simple at-home ways to tell if your lung function is maintaining its youthful levels. I believe exercising 5 minutes each hour throughout the day keeps you in the safe zone for the right amount of exercise so you will greatly optimize your energy production. And greater energy production results in less aging. Hundreds of studies show that people who exercise properly have lower rates of heart disease, cancer, diabetes, etc., and consistent movement and work from sunrise to sunset is how the farmer of older times stayed healthy and fit.

Feel Better, Look Better, Live Longer

Yes, you can literally REVERSE the aging process…even if you're already in your 50's, 60's, 70's, and 80's. At an age when many of your peers are slowing down, you can be busier than ever, doing pretty much whatever you want without limiting yourself.

You can have increased energy, higher libido, and more stamina while developing stronger muscles, smoother skin, and a powerful immune system that resists illness and disease. You can wake up every morning well rested, refreshed, and ready to take on the world.

"Men do not quit playing because they grow old; they grow old because they quit playing." — Oliver Wendell Holmes

And now my tiny secret: Exercising 5 minutes each hour provides optimal comprehensive fitness activities for men and women who don't want to quit playing. Activities for the body and mind are enjoyed all day long and this is key to a vibrant and healthy life.

The three core elements in my anti-aging program are:
1.) Strength training to maintain lean muscle and bone density.
2.) Cardiovascular exercise for heart and lungs.
3.) Stretching to maintain flexibility and prevent injury.

Isn't it smart to support all of the body, not just a few parts? My 5 minutes each hour anti-aging exercise system is also as simple and straight forward as possible, easy to understand and implement, yet varied and interesting so you don't get bored or burned out.

You choose the exercise YOU enjoy most to keep your level of enthusiasm high. It helps you stay focused on your goal for a healthier life. Don't feel that you have to do a certain exercise or that if you fail to do some of them every day and every hour that you wont get the benefit of an anti-aging program. Do what you can fit into your schedule and add to it when you can. Consistency is more important than duration.

Recent studies suggest that too much sitting is as bad as too little exercise. The farmer of yesteryear knew this and he kept himself moving as long as the sun was up. You have to speed up your pulse at various times of the day to help ward off cardiovascular disease, diabetes, obesity, and other problems.

But muscular inactivity of one-hour or more, such as sitting behind a computer or watching television, could cancel out any benefits from even 30 minutes of continuous exercise. We are discovering that frequent local muscle contraction is more important that the intensity of exercise once a day. And just as our ancestral farmer understood, it is suggested today that we stay physically busy—at least 5 minutes per hour—and avoid sitting in one place too long. Climbing stairs or other simple activities for 5 minutes each hour may prevent the onset of metabolic syndrome: high blood pressure, abdominal obesity, insulin resistance.

*****

Anything Can Happen on a Farm — Part IV

Universal Natural Health Care and Well-being. It used to *mean* something. It used to be a commitment between the farmer and his plants and animals. A solemn pledge that if he worked hard to take good care of them, they would give him all he needed for a fruitful life. But the modern big city has lost the wholesome consciousness of farming and has become nothing more than a cash cow for greed and self-indulgence supporting small retail/big corporate business and political government agencies. As a result, when we are born into city life we become handcuffed into a lifestyle living in fear and flirting with emotional disaster by choosing cheap sensual gratification over spiritual enrichment. Nothing proves this more than our feverish gift buying which has replaced the solemn religious holiday of Christmas.

As a result of peer pressure and overwhelming advertising and marketing psychology, a lot of truly conscientious and concerned people have trouble making lifestyle choices other than what profit-driven mainstream recommends…many of which could actually *make you sick!*

For the longest time, I was one of these vulnerable chumps, until I stood up and said "Enough now!"

I broke free from the money-driven comedy of modern city life and started to really live life again…

I dumped the typical mindset of the 40 hour work week with one 30-60 minute workout every other day…to help you live longer and healthier. That's why I set up this website. I discovered an incredibly effective and cheap alternative to the typical urban jungle fitness program which I believe can be life saving and too important to keep under wraps.

So I'm ready to crush the disinformation that mainstream is force-feeding you…and blow the doors off fake solutions to a wholesome life! My breakthrough secret passed one of the toughest tests — it works for me — and now I'm offering it to you so that within 6 weeks you can have…

**A Surge of All-Day Energy Like
Nothing You've Experienced…**

A Truly Changed Life!

The key to better health, fitness, and improved quality of life is to change the rules...

You change the rules...YOU win!

I pulled back the curtain and uncovered the most practical solution to a wholesome life that you may never hear about from your own doctor or fitness trainer. I'm now more relaxed, sleep better, think clearly, remember things better, and my mind is sharper. From my experience using this technique, I now believe that both YOU and I can become "Ageless Wonders" who never seem to get sick nor grow old. *And it just doesn't get easier than setting aside 5 minutes of your time, on average, every hour of your day.* It works for me and I'm sure it'll work for YOU too!

How is this possible?

Your mind can unlock the potent, incredible power within you...PROVEN...to improve your life...and wastes no time in Super-charging all of your cells — physical and mental bundles of work station powerhouses — to support your natural birthright to a wholesome blissful existence. And all it takes is *teeny little 5 minute breaks* scattered throughout your day.

The basic principle in my program rests on the developing field of epigenetics which states that traits acquired during your life, non-genetic variations, can be passed down through successive generations. Epigenetic inheritance examines how the environment influences the cellular level. The classic dramatic example was first presented by naturalist Jean Baptiste Lamarck and his giraffe. Lamarck concluded that when giraffes reached higher into the trees to munch on leaves, their necks became slightly longer — a trait variation that was passed on to descendants so that generation after generation of giraffes inherited slightly longer necks with the result we now see today.

We as humans can make conscious decisions which, due to the mind-body connection, will immediately set forth a chain reaction of energetic chemical processes that are driven to actually engineer the mental picture we create. By focusing on our picture day after day, the imagined idea will soon become... REAL.

Yet the giant gym rats aren't talking about this phenomenon, much less even thinking about it, and keep their treadmills running in overdrive...

They aren't saying a word about it because if their members discover that the mind is capable of creating perfect fitness and happiness, and this trait can be *passed on to their children,* the $14 billion a year physical fitness industry is going to implode!

I know this to be true and that's why I developed the quickest, easiest, and healthiest way to unlimited health and happiness... especially for people like YOU and ME that want to become REAL PEOPLE again... and is it ever effective!

*****

Anything Can Happen on a Farm — Part V

I'm fairly certain that for thousands of years my European descendants, and probably yours, were farmers. Recent research suggests that the men of Europe are descended from farming populations that migrated into Europe 10,000 years ago from the "Fertile Crescent", which stretches from Egypt across the Middle East into present-day Iraq. That's why I believed my agricultural genetic background PLUS epigenetic inherited traits would be paramount to help me change into a better human being — without having to leave the city and buy a farm.

Successful life on a farm depends on a strong 24/7 work ethic supported by a firm purpose driven conviction to understand the wholeness of nature. It came to me that all I had to do was incorporate those 2 principles into my daily life and still maintain a normal, but slightly adjusted, presence in modern society.

Before I go further, don't jump to conclusions and even think of giving up your job, income level, or friends... and plant a green garden... and you don't have to dress and act like a "new age freak." Keep the details of this new "experiment" to yourself and just make one slightly different change in the new you...

...and start living the life YOU want without compromise!

There is only one change — mental and physical — you have to make to get this to work, guaranteed, for you:

- **Focus — determined and consistent.**
- **Exercise or stretch for 5 minutes of every hour of waking day (as best you can).**

The details I am now sharing through this website, is that yesterday's enlightened farmer new what it took to stay healthy, prosperous, and satisfied with life. The day I realized how to use epigenetics to my benefit, I awakened the farming traits passed down to me over hundreds of generations, and I started taking my "virtual farm" with me everywhere I traveled. I now have a cow, pig, foal, and lowly snake to care for and they require my wholehearted attention for 5 minutes of every hour of every day, sunrise to sunset. During these short 5 minute time-outs from my personal and business work schedule I exercise or stretch with my animal friends to stay healthy with the purpose of eventually understanding the wholeness of the universe.

My virtual farm has become a worthy weapon to combat the vicious conspiracy designed to keep me sick, physically and spiritually... and it is effectively working in ways I never imagined!

I'm not telling you to drop the barbells, aerobics, yoga, tai chi, karate, kung fu, and any other dance you might be enjoying. All I'm saying is that to stay focused on the goal it takes consistent physical and mental attention and active work at least several minutes each hour during the day. And all you need to do is manage your schedule to allow short 5 minute breaks every hour.

The front lines of the fitness industry advertise that what you need to do is workout 20-40 minutes once a day or at least 3 times a week. I'm here to shout loudly that...

...IT DON'T WORK!

It doesn't work on a farm and it positively does not work in the city. Sure, people are getting bigger, stronger, and faster but the evidence shows the average fitness nut is not really getting **healthier, happier, or grasping a true feeling for the wholeness of nature.** I believe you must challenge the old ways of thinking about life, health, and fitness... not just follow in the rut and continue a system that isn't giving real valued results. And the only way to do this, in my opinion, is to tap into the original farming lifestyle, listen for the rooster crow, and remind yourself every hour to take care of the REAL business of life.

Very simple... and you don't have to change a thing about your life except... the focus of your attention... and a teeny bitty adjustment in your daily schedule. And your friends and associates will respect, maybe even imitate, you for your strong display of commitment to a self-improvement workout schedule,

I wouldn't PANIC if you have to skip a session here and there. This isn't supposed to break you. It should actually reduce stress in your life by setting goals that give you more focus and solid results with a feeling of control over the circumstances surrounding your life. Don't worry! When you get in-your-face results you will...

Anything Can Happen On A Farm   337

- Revive your drive...
- Lower your stress...
- Improve your health...
- Become more satisfied with life!

The problem with today's "once daily workout" is that after you shower your mind gets disconnected from the intention of better health. The rest of the day is focused on everything except the goal of wholeness. How can you be a part of the growing "Holistic" health movement if most of your day's awareness is on everything but the "whole?" You can't section out of your day a 30-60 minute workout and expect to get the same results as you would by focusing your mind consistently every hour... and the mind is a *very powerful force* for change. And I'm not telling you to give up your usual hardy workout, but to add just a teeny bitty more muscular activity throughout the day.

I'm convinced that by following this program you will slash your risk of metabolic syndrome, gain victory over your health and fitness, and you'll thank your lucky stars for the miracle of your life.

And no, I don't have any studies to back this up. It's a completely new idea and you are the first to hear about my personal experiment and results, but it makes good old fashion common sense. And yes, there has been some current research in the mental benefits of 5 minutes of "green exercise" done daily: {*http:// esciencenews.comarticles2010/05/01in.green.health.just5.minutes. green.exercise.optimal.good.mental.health*}

which backs up my own findings on the physical benefits of dispersing 5 minutes of physical exercise throughout the day.

By "farming" 5 minutes every hour, in addition to your usual workout, you will typically go through several stages:

1.) Total disbelief that only 5 minutes of exercise every hour can do so much.
2.) Rhetorical (and sometimes hostile) questioning and ridicule.
3.) Reading the information in this website again and reluctantly understanding it.
4.) Taking a leap of faith and starting the program with your own "virtual farm."
5.) Being highly impressed with the results.
6.) Becoming a "virtual farmer" enthusiast and trying to persuade friends.
7.) Being ignored and ridiculed by the friends who think you've lost your mind.
8.) After 3 months of tending your virtual farm animals your friends admiring the better physical look and condition you have.
9.) You telling them (again) that you exercise 5 minutes each and every hour possible in addition to your usual workout.
10.) Those friends reluctantly try virtual farming for 90 days. They repeat the above cycle from steps 5 on down.

*****

Anything Can Happen on a Farm — Part VI

Testosterone on Steroids? Is this what I'm talking about? NO WAY! Short term anabolic steroid use actually inhibits testosterone production and that is definitely not part of my game plan.

It might seem like I'm expressing a bulging, overactive, testosterone injected muscle head of male opinions, but nothing can be further from the truth. Most people think of testosterone as the difference between a soft cuddly-purring kitten and the more powerful focused, fearless, and determined wild tiger. These certainly are attributes that result from an optimal level of testosterone coursing through muscled veins, but the balanced titers of both testosterone and estrogen in a man and woman saturates each with a quiet, non-arrogant confidence, a confidence that results in an ego that's difficult to ding.

Think of the personality of the silverback male ape. As a rule he's usually very laid back, playing with the kids, but capable of incredible ferocity when challenged by another male. As soon as the challenger gives up, however, he stops — as if to say, "Good. You learned your lesson and don't do that again." He doesn't continue to fight as if he were still angry. He's not mean and testosterone does not make men mean. It's the imbalance between testosterone and estrogen levels that make men and women angry and mean.

My purpose is not to create a race of heartless aggressive beings, but to bring harmonious heartfelt balance to life through the free expression of instinct energy.

And in ending my FINAL question is:

**What's the fastest way
to learn what I'm presenting?**

**ACT
LIKE A
BABY**

and then

GO BABY, GO!

It's not the advice you'd expect. Learning a new skill can be a challenge, but unlearning and erasing a deeply embedded message might seem impossible as we recall from years of combat with our sugar addiction. Yet infants and children are born into a veritable jambalaya, figuring out the best behavioral responses purely from the sounds, objects, and interactions around them.

Their senses spark neural circuits that send stimuli to different areas of the brain matrix which opens up instinct driven energy meridians of the body.

These characteristics of the learning process are crucial for success:

First, and most importantly, a child's natural learning ability emerges only in an immersion environment free of verbal explanations.

Second, a child's learning is dramatically accelerated by constant feedback from family and friends. Positive correction and persistent reinforcement nurture the child's behavioral skill into full action-reaction expression.

Third, children learn through play. All the banter cavorting through young children's play with parents and playmates helps children develop behavioral skills that connect them to the world.

Adults possess this same powerful learning ability that orchestrated our success as children. Sadly, our clashes with "adult" society disarm our natural ability to think, act and instinctually respond appropriately to external stimuli forcing us to conclude that living free to relearn and express our natural instincts is hopeless. We simply don't have the instinct gene.

But I believe otherwise. You can recover your natural learning ability and set free your innate instinct to survive by prompting your brain to learn how to release the energetic flow of instinct the way it's wired to to your reflexes by complete immersion. My book gives you a method that does just that.

**_Teeth In Mortal Combat_ unlocks the
innate instinct learning ability
you acquired before birth and
master as a child.**

By recreating with baby steps the immersion context in which you learned your first proper response to outside stimuli, you will understand and react with confidence to life's challenges without relying on rules imprinted in your mind by society.

At every step and in every situation, you receive the correct feedback that prepares you for any imminent threat to your well-being.

**Your "instinct brain" remembers.
I have seen it in my own life.**

Act like a baby? You bet! Find out how you can reactivate your own innate, free flowing energy of instinct with _Teeth In Mortal Combat_. Then you'll be able to sleep like a baby, free of worries about your current and future challenges.

Scientists have identified a protein in breast milk that is DIRECTLY LINKED to blissful sleep in the infant…something "switches you off," relaxing your mind and body naturally for easy, deep, satisfying sleep.

Don't wait another 10 years for mainstream martial artists to catch on. You can sleep like a baby starting today. Let _Teeth In Mortal Combat_ be your "relaxation protein" for whatever ails you by helping you unleash your basic instinct for survival.

WHAT'S Holding YOU BACK?

While everyone is focusing on getting stronger and faster through specialized speed and strength clinics, there is new evidence that something else is causing loss of power and quickness with aging. And some experts believe that...

Chemical changes in the aging brain are what *really* cause diminished martial arts ability.

But that's only part of the equation. A tree is only as strong as its trunk and chi or energy flow is the trunk that supports all the chemical reactions in the body. If we search deeper, it is disturbances in the free flow of energy from the root system to the trunk that is even more revealing. And it is the negative taboos of society that twist and knot a matrix of clogging muck within the arterial system of our roots.

The REAL key is to be smarter — not stronger.

The key to the magical powers of martial arts is not to increase training time with harder exercises, but to increase the flow of primitive innate energy that has been held back by society's indiscriminate use of taboos.

Maximize your "deep" energy
AND boost muscle and brain power.

And much to my surprise, the greatest improvements in my personal martial arts skills appeared when I spent more of my time in deep meditation and focus on my teeth, jaw and tongue.

Scientists have a new respect for how the position and exercise of teeth, jaw and tongue affect the flow of nutrient rich blood and oxygen to the brain. The more ideal the jaw is positioned and the more exercise they engage in, the bigger is the performance of brain functions.

Now YOU know the...

Secret Weapon NOT Found
In 99.99% of Martial Arts Schools,
Seminars, Classes and Training Manuals

Everyone is hyping about the benefits of fancy kettle bells, traditional ropes and computerized exercise machines, yet they are missing out on one tiny detail. Negative Taboos wipe out the unbounded potential of the human mind and you'll never reach your full potential playing with these expensive fitness toys unless you can break free of the invisible grip society has on you.

So why isn't your teacher or coach telling you how to break free using the teeth, tongue and jaws? Simple, because they don't know and if they do know they aren't telling because it's too dangerous and much easier to sell expensive equipment, seminars, and memberships to fancy clubs, or worse yet, cheap dirty dojos.

This isn't really news, just a sad fact.

The well established schools of the martial arts world have big bucks riding on yesterday's answers. They don't care that their cash cows are outdated as long as they continue to get rich.

TRANSLATION: They will soon start covering up my new research that proves their old training theories and systems are like a Benjamin Franklin key on a kite compared to a Large Hadron Collider.

So the schools will continue to push their ineffective teachings and their marketing managers will want to downplay my new discovery that make their solutions, if not obsolete, at least watered down.

As a result, unless you read my book, you'll most likely be wasting a lot of money on inferior products and STILL feel like sick, tired, old and incompetent as a martial artist.

With my book, you can help solve problems that society creates for you and begin laying the foundation for good health and a happy life. That is why it's one of the most important books on the market to date. Don't suffer any longer!

The Entire Field of Martial Arts Should Be Re-Evaluated in Light of This New Breakthrough Book

Instinct is the miraculous natural guide to healing...

Struggling self-defense skills
Murky sluggish metabolism
Fading memory and mental performance
Low libido
Degenerating arteries and heart trouble
Tumor Growth
Normal blood sugar
Losing life span
Timid cellular immunity
"Bad luck"
Poor judgment

**When you have sharp instincts
you feel more alive in every way.**

Too Little Instinct Flowing Through Your Meridians? Some Would Say You're As Good As Drunk

You are an accident waiting to happen. Even minor disturbances in your instinct can cause you to experience momentary bouts of being zoned out from the world around you. It's almost as if you are sleepwalking, except you are awake, not asleep! Your brain starts to shut down.

**No instinct, no energy.
No energy, no life!**

Please, dear friend, don't let this happen to you!

Teeth In Mortal Combat helps you **"Switch On"** day after day for a life of satisfying health and wellness, PLUS, you'll feel more secure in your surroundings whether at home, work or on your way to the store. You'll feel stronger and younger because your whole body will be energized with a freer flow of energy.

And when your body is flooded with energy, you feel *incredibly renewed* ... and can get back to enjoying life's pleasures as nature intended.

Order your copy of my book today to discover the healing miracle of your teeth, tongue and jaws. This discovery has worked for me and I'm convinced that *Teeth In Mortal Combat* will be a Godsend for you.

It will be the best thing you've done for your self in years!

Your for health, longevity and emotional security!

Lester Sawicki, D.D.S.

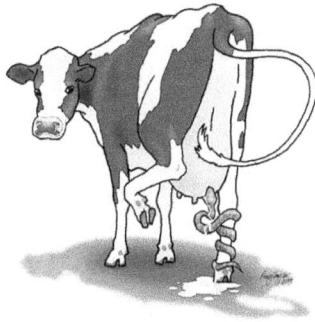

END BONUS CHAPTERS: PART 1
TEETH IN MORTAL COMBAT

Bite, Chew, Eat... and Carry A Bright Belly

—*from the TAO TE TOOTH*

The
Teeth
Whitening
Cure

A HOLISTIC GUIDE TO
BRIGHT SMILES AND
BETTER HEALTH
IN A TOXIC
WORLD

LESTER SAWICKI, DDS

The Teeth Whitening Cure

*Bonus Chapters
44 through 51*

Chapter 44
TEETH SENSE WHITENING

"Exhilarating" new SMILE breakthrough will have you smiling bright…in the best way possible!"

Dear Seekers of Better and Safer Teeth Whitening,

No one likes to talk about it, but let's face it, as we get older, it's often the first thing to go. You know what I mean—that certain glow…the one that happens when you SMILE. And the glamour industry leads us to believe the glow…that pure sexy radiance portrayed in Hollywood…can be painted into a person by a simple cosmetic makeover with teeth whitening.

But the worst part is, we accept their half-truths. And after your complete makeover, when the quality of your life takes a nose dive, it makes your whole life a lot less pleasurable and your bank account a whole lot thinner.

But what if it didn't have to be that way? Imagine how much better your life would be if you could get back the kind of innocent glowing smile you owned as a teenager…with all the health and energy that went along with it. Wouldn't you give anything to own that magic again?

That's why I wrote the breakthrough book, *The Teeth Whitening Cure*, that not only solves the problem, it also lets you enjoy the best days of your life!

The Teeth Whitening Cure is THE Right Solution

Sure, store shelves are full of teeth whitening products—from simple toothpastes to complicated gel trays and strips. But unlike all of the other choices, my discovery doesn't only work on getting teeth whiter…it actually enhances the whole oral health experience, and makes fully energized living better and better.

And while other dentists may focus only on bleaching yellow teeth—which really does happen as we get older—that's not the only factor affecting a sexy smile. "Vigorous" health is the other half of the equation for a radiant smile.

The best smile starts in your brain

If your teeth are white, but your heart and mind just aren't in the mood, you might have an adequate smile…but it won't be **great.** Stress, disease, and less than vigorous health will detract from your performance and enjoyment of a glamorous smile.

It turns out there's a much better way to fire up your winning smile…and experience long-lasting-passionate smiles and the most satisfying enjoyment of life you've ever felt.

A complete oral health renewing game plan

In *The Teeth Whitening Cure* you'll discover chapters that focus on the aging process…and pearls of wisdom and advice on how to stop, stall, and reverse it. No other book on the market reveals…Secrets to Healthy Teeth Whitening.

The tip of the iceberg

Yellow teeth and a discolored tongue are what I call a "tip of the iceberg" condition. That's because discolored teeth may be just a surface issue complicated by something deeper in a discolored tongue—there are a wide variety of metabolic disorders and other serious health conditions that can set the stage for discolored teeth and tongue:

infections

medications

nutritional deficiencies
anemia
bleeding disorders
complications of pregnancy
diminished salivary output due to obstructions, radiation
    therapy, chemotherapy
metal poisoning
antibiotic misuse
fluoride poisoning
Sjorgen's Syndrome
extreme high or low body temperature

It's a proven fact your teeth and tongue can give you a more complete picture of your overall health. That's why I've written the ONLY book on HOW to whiten teeth in a more holistic way. So that you can be aware of the various reasons why your teeth and tongue might be discolored in the first place. And then take action—see your medical doctor and dentist for a thorough evaluation of your condition—and then take the necessary safe steps to whiten your teeth in a *Healthier Way.*

The search for *real* pain relief finally ends

...When the pain from laser teeth whitening reaches cursing level, you don't have to try endless ineffective bleach solutions... an exhaustive search that will end up in vain. *The Teeth Whitening Cure* is the remedy that will bring pain down *Fast* from agonizing to barely a whisper.

American dentists have found that 2 out of 3 bleaching patients report mild and transient tooth sensitivity. Some people experience intolerable sensitivity and must stop the treatments. This is especially more common with the newer laser bleach treatments found in upscale cosmetic dental offices.

The Teeth Whitening Cure shows you a more painless, holistic approach to whitening teeth that really works…and it works **safely.** The holistic remedies in the breakthrough book work because they tackle all of the problems of laser teeth bleaching: the unbearable symptoms and the underlying causes, PLUS, it even shows you how to repair the damage laser bleaching can unleash on your enamel and minimize dangerous side effects.

The best way I know how to take the suffering of laser teeth whitening down from "cursing level" to barely a whisper is to just—DON'T DO IT! Follow the holistic guidelines in my book and you'll be smiling pain free again!

Chapter 45
HAVE A WHITER SMILE AND GET HEALTHY TOO

**Would YOU Like to LOOK and FEEL
Like a Healthy 25 Year Old?**

**Lose Yellowing Stains.
Regain Energy.
Have More Self-confidence.**

"You can restore your natural magnetic Smile Power to that of a Healthy 25 Year Old with The Teeth Whitening Cure."

**Is this book great or what?
Your Natural Born Smile Becomes A
Canvas of Mother Nature's Artwork.**

Imagine your smile transformed into a bright beautiful, meaningful, and easy work of art just like mother nature intended.

Isn't it time to make your inner and outer smile outstanding?
Give The Gift Of A Naturally Bright Smile.

Help a loved one by surprising them with a copy of the one and only... *The Teeth Whitening Cure.*

A Different Kind of Yellow Teeth Relief

**THIS BOOK COULD
SAVE THE SMILE
OF YOUR LOVED ONE**

356 The Teeth Whitening Cure — *Bonus Chapters*

SIMPLE

Get all your soldiers in order and it takes only
 10–15 minutes.

SAFE

No toxic chemicals involved... food grade ingredients only.

RELIABLE

You're in total control.

No chance of painful cold sensitive teeth.

Ghost teeth? Won't happen after you read all about it.

AFFORDABLE

Stop Blowing Money!

Perfect Gift For GRADS and DADS!

The book costs $16.95. The revealed secrets are priceless.

Are Your Teeth Whitening Products Working FOR or AGAINST You?

Today's teeth bleaching manufacturers have become teeth bleaching hydrogen peroxide-dispensing assembly lines. They sell whatever the consumer will buy, regardless of whether it is effective or has questionable toxic chemicals. It is my mission to help you preserve your *health using naturally safe products and save you money all with the intention of improving your health.*

Does Your Bleaching Manufacturer Care
if You
Live or Die?

Finally! A Teeth Whitening System That Works
With Ingenious Answers To Genuine Concerns...
...Easy, Safe, Natural, Non-Toxic.

This rare book offers advice on the safety and effectiveness of teeth whitening products and how they can work synergistically with nutrients and supplements to keep you healthy.

So keep this in mind... **The Teeth Whitening Cure puts your welfare first.** It is a lower cost solution that may work better than expensive bleaching brand names. It also combines bleaching expertise with in-depth knowledge of potentially harmful chemical ingredients and oxidizing reactions. *The Teeth Whitening Cure* is committed to helping you get the very best results from teeth bleaching with a more natural and safer approach.

So if you want to get HEALTHY, DETOXIFY, and LOSE TOOTH STAINS...buy yourself a copy. Don't cheat yourself with ineffective and potentially toxic over-the-counter products. The Teeth Whitening Cure shows you how to achieve more natural results at home AND save money as well.

Beauty and the Bleach

Experience a lush abundance of natural beauty. Don't tell your smile it can't be naturally bright. Technology has given us 24/7 LIVES...and 24/7 STRESS. Can technology give us back a 24/7 natural smile? I invite you to learn about the science of natural teeth whitening. The book gives you support, education and tools you need to help enrich your smile and keep it glowing. It gives you something to smile about and is your 1st Class Ticket to organic smile health.

Reveal Your Inner Smile with a Little Outside Help

Connect With the Soul of Your Smile

Inner Beauty—Outer Sexy

It's a new year... and make it your best year ever with a copy of *The Teeth Whitening Cure*! This is the year that you make personal health and wellness a top priority—bringing focus and intention to your smile and fitness goals, being mindful of what you put into your mouth for whitening and fuel, and bringing your best energy to your daily life and those people that matter most to you. To support you in your journey, The Teeth Whitening Cure provides essential strategies for an oral and whole body wellness plan that is sure to bring results!

Remember: exercise and movement play a critical role in your smile health. A healthy smile is an active one! The Teeth Whitening Cure shows you how to combine all elements necessary to:

Reduce your hunger for "excessive" whitening.

Boost your energy, eliminate fatigue, burn more calories efficiently.

Strip away and detox unwanted yellow stains naturally and keep them off.

Achieve your long-term healthy smile goals.

Enhance your overall wellness for a lifetime.

This is probably the most significant teeth whitening guide you will ever read. It has a great story, explains things very clearly, and is sure to be exciting and useful. And if you have friends and loved ones...

Start Their Future With Something Magical.
Give them a copy of The Teeth Whitening Cure.

It's a holistic guide to minimally invasive at-home teeth bleaching treatments so you can show off your gorgeous teeth again. And it will show you how to avoid suffering painful, cold sensitive teeth that you might have experienced after your dentist professionally applied his teeth bleaching formulas. Think of is as your *"comfort zone"* for teeth whitening.

For about the price of a decent dinner, the book offers a truly unique, customizable system for bleaching that can be fine tuned for your teeth. Bleach more efficiently—**see and feel the difference.** After all…

…if all teeth are different,
why are all teeth whitening products
virtually the same?

Get The Teeth Whitening Cure NOW!
Learn how the power of natural attraction brings you
FREE smiles!

CHAPTER 46
BEYOND BLEACHING

By now I'm sure you've seen quite a few ads for teeth bleaching. With good reason. It's discovery over 30 years ago was a major breakthrough at the forefront of cosmetic dentistry—one that yields astonishing results for your yellowing smile and quality of life.

But...

You cannot be satisfied with simply the latest fad—no matter how good it is. You deserve and should demand more. In other words, teeth bleaching by itself is NOT a magic bullet.

That's where my book, *The Teeth Whitening Cure,* comes in. I show you how combining teeth bleaching with detox can **enhance and empower your body's ability to heal itself.** It's that powerful. And urgent. It also makes good TEETH SENSE. That's the Winning Knock-Out Punch...a left and right hook my book introduces to you...whitening and detox. I've taken the good, examined it, and made it better. The formulas were developed to take you another step forward—with the keys to robust health and vitality...into your 80's, 90's and beyond.

Conventional teeth bleaching products are based on some science, but usually promote magical and wishful thinking. They lack any real substance nor hope to increase your health and well being.

Wishful thinking is fun and can be a creative exercise that allows you to visualize the future, contemplate unlimited possibilities, and actually begin to attract a new reality to you.

But if you allow yourself to be led with magical promises advertised by money-hungry teeth whitening companies, you're likely to invite a negative future with apocalyptic health events looming on the horizon.

Here's something most people don't know...

The Future of Optimal Health and Life-Extension is Here, Now...

... and it begins with bleaching your yellowing teeth in a Healthy Way.

Hydrogen peroxide is the primary bleaching agent used to whiten teeth. It penetrates and unclogs the tooth enamel, traveling through microscopic tubes all the way to the nerve pulp. It is generally believed that the small amount reaching the tooth nerve does no permanent harm to a healthy nerve pulp, but how certain can you be that your nerve is healthy?

Medical doctors often say an athlete's heart is healthy only to tragically find that person fall dead during game time. Unfortunately, your dentist's evaluation of your tooth nerve health can fall short just like your medical doctor's heart tests. So, if you bleach it is wise to support your tooth pulp with good nutrition and antioxidant therapy in order to help prevent nerve damage.

Hydrogen peroxide, however, when used outside of "cosmetic" bleaching can increase good health and has a long history of success. The Teeth Whitening Cure is the only book that examines the healthy use of hydrogen peroxide therapy during teeth bleaching.

Oxygen is our most prevalent and abundant nutrient, yet the most overlooked one. We can literally live for months without food, days without water, but only minutes without oxygen. Your tooth needs oxygen and unless it is well oxygenated you cannot hope to have teeth in optimal health. The internal blood vascular system supplies your tooth with oxygen and exercise with oxygen therapy (EWOT) is one of the easiest ways to bring oxygen to your tooth pulp. Hydrogen peroxide swished orally and applied during teeth bleaching is one of the best ways to soak the outside surface of your tooth with an abundance of oxygen.

FINALLY SOME GOOD NEWS!! Optimal oxygen in the body and tooth gives vigorous health and vitality at the *SPEED-OF-LIGHT*. Well-oxygenated cells do not get sick. Extra oxygen, or supersaturation, can give you more energy and allow a calmer feeling of peace. Super-oxygenation with ozone is now being used in dentistry to help heal cavities.

Oxygen treatment in the right concentration and amount has no negative side effects. It actually enhances the healing process. It improves and restores the immune system and may be the most significant single factor in preventing illness. The beneficial use of hydrogen peroxide and it's transfer of oxygen to the tooth during teeth bleaching is what *The Teeth Whitening Cure* is all about.

Since 1920 there are well over six thousand articles in science publications about hydrogen peroxide. Thousands of doctors in Europe, Scandinavia, the United States and Mexico are using it successfully to treat degenerative disease. *The Teeth Whitening Cure* will convince you that there are dental as well as medical benefits to bleaching your teeth with hydrogen peroxide—as long as it is done in a healthy way...

> **...And mainstream teeth whitening companies DO NOT understand what it means to whiten teeth in a "healthier way."**

That's where *The Teeth Whitening Cure* comes in...

> *...How to get the benefits of "increased health" during teeth bleaching.*

CHAPTER 47
TWO SUPER BOWL WINNERS

Introducing Two Super Bowl Winners
That Can Engineer Health and Wellness...
Teeth Bleaching and Detox

Dear Teeth Whitening Friend,

Harvard Research, Nobel Prize Research, and Powerful Antioxidants Jump Start Teeth Whitening to a New Level.

Enjoy a miraculous new life!

Anti-Aging Miracle—DETOX—is Here Today!

Guess what?

What was science fiction 30 years ago is here, now. And you don't have to be young to enjoy the benefits. In fact, a Teeth Whitening Detox is considered a Godsend for Baby Boomers.

Thanks to these two amazing processes—bleaching and detox—people all over are reporting vigorous health...amazing turnarounds...and "super-human" smiles. Even people who've had less than perfect oral hygiene all their lives.

And the answers are available to you, right now.

Let me introduce myself. My name is Dr. Lester Sawicki. As a dentist, I've cared for over 100,000 patients in my 30+ years of practice. I've seen how poor dental health can ravage the mouth and body. And I've seen how the right combination of teeth bleaching and organ detox can change your life.

Can You Imagine a Day When
Your Biggest Health Fears Are Banished By These
Two Revolutionary Solutions?

That day has arrived!

I don't believe in magic bullets. I believe in sound, solid science. That's why I wrote the book, *The Teeth Whitening Cure,* to finally reveal to you... Secrets to Healthy Teeth Whitening and Detox.

If it sounds too good to be true... rest assured. The Teeth Whitening Cure will convince you of the amazing benefits of "healthy" teeth bleaching and detox.

Ancient Remedy Even More Powerful

Over 4000 years ago the ancient medicinal book of the Hindus described the use of urine therapy to be one of their most powerful medicinal treatments for many types of disease. According to some sources, it may well be the most researched and most medically proven natural remedy. Urine therapy was practiced in Greece and they also used it to bleach and whiten their teeth.

Today's science has switched from urine to hydrogen peroxide for even *more powerful results*. Hydrogen peroxide, either used for teeth bleaching or as an internal detoxing cure, works similarly to urine—only better.

Our sun is the "Great Purifier." Its ionizing rays produce hydrogen peroxide (H_2O_2) in the atmosphere that helps cleanse the air of pollutants. Likewise, when we inhale nebulized hydrogen peroxide mist, the H_2O_2 cleanses our lungs, sinuses, throat, bronchial tract— areas most affected by viruses—by killing infected cells that are functioning as viral laboratory workshops. When used correctly, this natural therapeutic weapon of mass destruction cannot fail to wipe out all types of viral infections, and it does so without side effects. This "great purifier" burns away many toxic substances found on the internal and external surfaces of our bodies. We need only discover and unleash the science behind nature's cure for disease.

In my teeth whitening system, hydrogen peroxide is the chemical that bleaches stains out of teeth. I believe the safe, healthy use of hydrogen peroxide can not only whiten teeth, but also detoxify the body of impurities. In fact, it was a team of periodontists working to cure gum disease who discovered the teeth whitening "side- effect" of hydrogen peroxide.

Fortunately it is not necessary to drink hydrogen peroxide (the ancients drank urine) in order to receive its health-promoting components as they are easily absorbed into the highly vascular oral mucosa when just rinsing with it. While rinsing, the peroxide travels through oral tissues into the body's circulatory network and thereby exerts its holistic, disease-curing effect.

CHAPTER 48
SHOCKING RESULTS

**Top Echelons of Scientific Research
Unveil Shocking Results:
Life-extension: 30-60%!**

Researchers found ways to extend lifespan in the following species: Yeast, by 60%, worms, by 30%, fish, by 60%.

Life extension occurs when certain enzymes are triggered.

Studies on humans have shown that you can trigger similar enzymes, however, there is no proof that humans receive the same life extension benefits as yeast, worms, and fish. We do know that calorie restriction and certain nutritional extracts switch on these enzymes which then trigger "survival" genetic pathways that lower blood pressure, enhance fat metabolism, improve blood sugar levels, cleanse heart and liver tissues and increase insulin sensitivity.

Your body then acts like a younger leaner, stronger you.

Pharmaceutical companies are trying to develop drugs that trigger life extension pathways and there is hope for success within the next five years. We all know, however, that drugs usually have side effects that are worse than the symptoms, and this should cause one to be suspicious of any chemical pill sold as a *fountain of youth.*

The closest science has come to a true fountain of youth, without drugs, occurred in the early 1900's when Dr. Alexis Carrel, of the Rockefeller Institute for Medical Research performed an amazing experiment on the heart cell of a chicken embryo.

He managed to sustain the life of the chicken cells by immersing them in a solution containing all the nutrients necessary for life and detoxing the excreted waste solution daily. This is called "cleaning house'" by taking out the trash. The average chicken lives only about 7 years while the detoxed chicken heart embryo cells survived 29 years.

Can a detox reverse a lifetime of poor diet health risks?

Conventional medicine claims a detox has no medical use, at least not the kind of detox mainstream physicians are familiar with. This means most mainstream medical doctors won't prescribe a detox for you such as:

> fasting with pure water and juices
> cleansing diets made up of less alcohol and refined/processed foods
> herbal internal organ support
> vitamin/mineral/food extracts that chelate heavy metals
> hydrogen peroxide and healing clay baths
> ...and the list goes on.

The problem arises because medical insurance will not pay for a detox unless it is related with an alcohol/drug addiction or the patient has compromised liver pathways necessary to properly metabolize chemical drugs such as:

> aspirin
> acetaminophen found in Tylenol
> ibuprofen found in Advil
> non steroidal anti-inflammatory drugs such as Celebrex
> anti-anxiety drugs such as Valium, Prozac

(Dentists have this same problem with insurance. We know how to prevent cavities by helping the patient control salivary phi, but most dental insurance companies will not pay for the simple, common sense diagnostic test.)

Cutting edge researchers, not handcuffed with mainstream insurance politics, have shown that liver/kidney detox pathways can be improved by sweating through exercise and heat saunas, plus taking vitamins, minerals, herbs, and antioxidants either internally or applied externally to improve the detoxification of:

> Pollution in the air we breathe, x-ray radiation, electromagnetic fields, etc.
> Pesticides
> Drugs
> Chemicals in our food and water supply
> Household and personal care products
> Negative thoughts and emotions

These toxins are contributing to illness and disease in our world. And while its impossible to avoid toxic substances completely, you can help your body expel them with regular detoxification. This is especially important if your own organ detox pathways are not functioning at peak levels.

Aging occurs when various cellular and molecular systems decline in function. These changes are influenced by genetics, metabolism, and environment. In younger people, cell damage from the toxic sludge of normal metabolism can be repaired. Aging organisms that lose their ability to repair usually have a major decline in the cells ability to remove the trash. "Cleaning house", as in detoxing, was the single reason the embryo chicken heart kept beating for 29 years and it should also add years to our quality of life.

The main organs of detoxification are lungs, liver, colon, kidneys, and skin. After years and years of toxic overload and then suppressing your body's own natural cleansing cycle, your major organs will simply give up the struggle and become "diseased." Your body, lacking the life-force to fight, will then succumb to fatigue and illness. Supporting your elimination organs as they age, before the breakdown, make sense.

Cautions About Detoxification

Extreme detox protocols are appropriate only when toxicity is confirmed and verified. Assumptions that we are toxic because we live in a toxic environment are generally incorrect according to Traditional Chinese Medicine. When the body is harmonious, it cleanses itself remarkably well. Purgation therapies, though they may improve symptoms temporarily, rarely solve long term problems, because they do not address root causes. Even more dangerous is the fact that detox therapies are usually costly to the Qi and many complaints that motivate people to detox are actually caused by weak Qi.

And that is why *The Teeth Whitening Cure* was written, to reveal this and much more information vital to your health when you undertake teeth bleaching.

How to prepare your body for the potentially harmful creation of free radicals when hydrogen peroxide bursts onto the scene.

How free radicals are a critical component of bleaching and how to create better balance between harmful and helpful free radicals during the bleach process.

And how and when to incorporate a teeth detox, if needed.

Remember, teeth breathe, sweat, and detox just like the rest of your body and when you bleach with hydrogen peroxide it pays to know the details for your overall health and the health of your teeth.

Why Not Just Start Bleaching the Healthier Way, Now?

You don't have to be an elite athlete to enjoy a leaner you with a greatly enhanced aerobic capacity. Bleach wisely and your muscles will be consuming oxygen more efficiently because they'll have healthier and greater numbers of mitochondria (and thus a greater capacity to generate energy.) Bleach without knowing all the facts, and hydrogen peroxide bursting into the tooth and oral cavity has the capacity to harm the cell walls of mitochondria, literally shutting down the energy grid inside your body.

What's the secret to getting more energy? Keeping the cell walls of your mitochondria intact and efficiently detoxing the waste from the water-protein matrix of enzymes within these little "powerhouse furnaces." That means if your main detox organs are not working efficiently or you overwhelm them with substances like teeth bleaching liquids, powders, gels, and strips, your could be severely stressing your mitochondria to the point of failure.

Your worst nightmare is now over!
You can assist and enhance the detox of the oral/whole body matrix with these amazing health benefits:

Boost energy and vitality

Replenish energy after bleaching, which depletes energy to some extent

Protect and rebuild tooth enamel and muscle

Fortify your body against aging, which depletes energy, brain, and heart cell life, and your ability to use energy to thrive

Improve your body's cellular defense against free radical attack

Every cell in your body contains mitochondria. Researchers know that healthy mitochondria can do more than just boost your energy level. They're the secret keys to a life that's active and vital into your 70's, 80's, 90's, and beyond.

The "dynamic duo" of teeth bleaching and detox can not only brighten your smile, but when done in a "healthier" way can give you an amazing BONUS...

...a Powerful Punch...
that can Raise Your Life Experience to a
Miraculous New Level of Joy and Prosperity!

Hurry NOW and get your valuable copy of
The Teeth Whitening Cure!

CHAPTER 49
BREAK ALL BARRIERS
TO BETTER HEALTH

News Alert!
The Teeth Whitening Cure
Breaks All Barriers to Better Health!

Cosmetic Teeth Bleaching + increased Physical Fitness
Gives You...
The Best Smile of Your Life!

Say goodbye to yellow teeth and low energy! Transcend all
the potential dangers of teeth whitening and thrive with "high energy" everyday... for life!

...with the one little <u>secret</u> that could free you... for good...

Finally, a teeth whitening protocol with answers for:

blood oxygenation
tip-top immune defenses against "body breakdown"
endless vigor until your very last breath!

Dentists say it's finally happening... discovered... important secrets to whitening teeth as well as improving health and
fitness... as you age, instead of watching life slip through your
fingers.

Now the secret's out and available to you in...

The Teeth Whitening Cure

Inside the pages of the little "everything" book, learn the science behind incredible revelations that could free you from all the dangers of a toxic world for the rest of your long healthy life!

Buy now to own the first ever book of its kind…look back to remember how many times you have heard it said…

"You just have to live with it."

Try saying that to someone struggling to bleach out the yellow—screaming with the acute pain of cold sensitive teeth… reaching for pain pills to dull the throbbing aches…or wracked with the struggle of getting through another day of low energy.

"Well, It Just Isn't So! If you want to live your best
(and I think you do) you'll want to know what
science shows is now possible:

Say goodbye to Yellow Teeth and Low Energy!

Most of us have no qualms with getting older. It's getting *old* that's the problem. Right when we start coming into our own—and finally enjoying what we've worked so hard for—is the time we're losing the wonderful attributes of youth…

Bright White Teeth
and an
Energy Spiked Enthusiasm

Our teeth begin to yellow and our once firm bodies soften, sag and drag. Our tongue, lips, and cheeks wrinkle and our razor edge senses slowly dull like an old limping hound dog. It's downright depressing.

But there's good news…
incredible discoveries have been made.

Geneticists have identified genes that could make us "ageless." Hard to believe, but true. So far they've been able to extend the lives of lab animals up to four times longer. Gerontologists and anti-aging researchers agree that normal life expectancy will reach 150, 300, even 1000 years within the next century...

Who wants to live longer when your body's
falling apart at the seams?

I think you'll agree, you want to be able to enjoy your days and nights full tilt! And if you're no longer silting to settle for looking older every year—with yellowing teeth—and feeling it too—you'll be happy to know...

Dentists, nutritionists, and fitness experts working together, have uncovered another breakthrough that can help you... renew your yellowing teeth to a more natural youthful bright white and...

Slow aging, improve your health
and fitness, retain your senses...
... and do it <u>right now</u>.

Outdated but still mainstream, conventional medicine will tell you that the rate at which you age is based almost entirely on your genetic makeup. In other words, the DNA you inherit from your parents has a unique genetic code which triggers when you'll lose your smarts, your senses, and your energy.

But while were waiting for geneticists to finish unraveling the mysteries of our DNA, the science of epigenetics is making headlines. It is a rapidly growing research field that investigates heritable alterations in gene expression caused by mechanisms other than changes in DNA sequence. In other words, by controlling your environment you can override your DNA triggers.

Epigenetics plus nutritional breakthroughs and exciting advances in exercise physiology are promising to change our lives for the better.

Enjoy the "good life"—no compromises—well into your 100's!

Not only can you look great, you can feel great too. You can naturally rejuvenate your body, organ by organ, cell by cell from top to bottom including your smile.

I reveal in my new book, tools and nutrients that are used in anti-aging centers around the world and the results are spectacular. When incorporated with good common sense, into a teeth whitening protocol, you can expect the same as reported from patients in these anti-aging centers:

Endless energy and strength
Brighter smiles
Superior memory
Fewer cavities
Sharp vision and hearing
Reversed gum disease
Solid heart health
Less wear and tear on the body
Longer life
Greater self-confidence
More success

Every cell in your body is powered by little batteries called *mitochondria*. They look like tiny dots under the microscope. Yet these 'batteries" literally generate much of your physical and *mental energy*.

The problem is teeth bleaching uses different complexes of hydrogen peroxide and the end result is an outburst of oxidative free radicals which breakdown mitochondrial cell membranes. The little batteries get "gunked up" and corrode like an old battery potentially leading to loss of endurance, less focus, wear and tear on the body, disease, and shorter life.

And that's where I take the bull by the horns in showing you how to safely use anti-oxidants during teeth bleaching to fight free radicals. Teeth bleaching then becomes safer and healthier than conventional methods used in most of today's dental offices and over the counter bleach systems.

But it's only the beginning as *The Teeth Whitening Cure* takes you continents away revealing little known secrets that restore youthful living to a point where:

> Teeth became more resistant to decay!
> Stress levels plummet!
> Performance levels soar!
> Gums revitalize!
> Folks get smarter!
> Hearts get stronger!

Plus, the unexpected miracle you never heard your dentist mention because this is cutting edge...

Get the age-fighting and smile-whitening breakthrough book now jam packed with health and fitness information... found only in *The Teeth Whitening Cure*!

While the research is still ongoing the science is suggesting that it is now possible to...

Safely tip control of your health back into your hands and teeth bleaching in a healthier way is a key factor favoring your success. That's why *The Teeth Whitening Cure* was written. To show you how to put the top researched powerhouses to work for you when you bleach your teeth whiter.

While no one is saying we'll all live to be 100 because of these discoveries (at least not yet!), today, we can enjoy every day we're given. Without the fear of losing youthful energy, fading memory, or any other "aging" worries that some say long term teeth bleaching contributes to.

Buy the book and start seeing the difference in the way you feel. Teeth bleaching, in a healthier way, can contribute added benefits to your quality of life in ways that your dentist might never had told you. The benefits can keep going and adding up so that, hopefully with time, you'll feel 35 years younger!

Be on your way to a healthy, happy, bright smiling
100 years plus!

Buy it now!
SPECIAL REPORT
TEETH WHITENING UPDATE:

For years, one teeth whitening puzzle has frustrated dentists around the globe, until now...

DENTIST breaks the "secret code" to the greatest teeth whitening challenge of our time!

Discover the NEW BREAKTHROUGH book...that has all the Secrets to Healthy Teeth Whitening...Revealed!

PLUS...
...The Perfect Cure for Bleach Fever!

Dear Friend in Search of Healthy Bright Teeth,

This is BIG. Dentists and their patients have been waiting for this moment for years.

It all started over 30 years ago when periodontal researchers were looking for a cure for gum disease. They decided to try applying hydrogen peroxide into diseased gum pockets because they new it attacked the many harmful bacteria associated with gum disease. To their surprise they noticed their test subject's tooth color was changing from yellow to white.

But there was one HUGE problem—It Worked Too Well!... and there were potential negative side effects...and they had to find a way to get their secret to work SAFELY for you.

You see, hydrogen peroxide used in teeth whitening creates potentially dangerous free radicals. It is the free radicals that damage mitochondria cell membranes that may be harmful to your health and even ultimately lead to Death.

But hydrogen peroxide works like magic to whiten teeth and throughout the world teeth bleaching has now become a feverish phenomenon. Teeth Whitening has reached world-wide pandemic proportions...and people everywhere have developed "bleach fever" in their rush to whiten teeth...to get a fix for that "Hollywood Smile."

The Teeth Whitening Cure is the NEW Breakthrough book that shows you how to fight free radical damage with healthy teeth whitening—like nothing else before it...

AND...it's the...

Perfect Cure for Bleach Fever!

Up until now the secrets to healthy teeth whitening has been puzzling dentists and their patients with three BIG hurdles:

Hurdle #1...SOLVED: most of the hydrogen peroxide on the market is unsafe to use orally. They have potentially hazardous stabilizers including acetanilide, phenol, sodium stagnate, and tertrasodium phosphate, much of which gets absorbed into your kidneys and liver through highly vascular gum, tongue, and cheek tissues.

Hurdle #2…SOLVED: free radicals can result in tissue damage, accelerated aging, degenerative disease, and likely involved in the development of cancer and/or the development of infectious diseases.

Hurdle #3…SOLVED: the vast majority of adverse events due to teeth whitening are reported as oral soft tissue irritation and tooth sensitivity. The reports range from "transient and mild" to "horrible throbbing toothache leading to migraine headaches."

But it is with great excitement that I introduce to you what could be the very best answer, in one incredible book, to all three of these puzzles…

The Teeth Whitening Cure
The ONLY CURE for…Bleach Fever!

The Teeth Whitening Cure is a BRAND NEW approach to teeth whitening. It is a HUGE victory for you—especially if you've tried bleaching without a hint of results in either brightening or increased health. It has all the possible answers to serious questions about the safety of teeth whitening…and once word gets out EXPOSING all the facts, it may very well become:

Your Soul Vaccination Against Bleach Fever

It is now <u>becoming the natural efficacious alternative to conventional teeth whitening the world has been waiting for</u>.

But there's EVEN MORE to this
revolutionary book…

The Teeth Whitening Cure is already providing you with answers to the potential dangers of teeth whitening, but I wanted to push it over the top!

So I added a healthy dose of information on:

support for STRONG teeth and bones
promoting a "cavity-free" life
maintaining Peak Physical Fitness

The book even goes one step further and includes a special chapter on "Black Tongue" to make sure you understand all its causes and solutions if it ever creeps into your life... from ancient superstitious mythology to hard scientific facts.

It is proven to have good results.

It is an effective and significant improvement over all the teeth whitening products on the market today...

and it just keeps getting better...

...so you can see why this unique revolutionary book had to be written... setting new standards for healthier classic teeth whitening... with all the talk of a toxic world becoming worse.

All of the research, the countless hours, the detailed studies have led to this...

Finally—teeth whitening for the 21st century!

Here it is: The NEW solution where Nothing has been left out—and nothing has been spared.

Rejuvenate your smile... with a new approach to promoting healthy teeth whitening results... AND—the bar was set HIGH-ER with the unique discoveries revealed.

...so what are you waiting for?

This is the NEWEST BREAKTHROUGH in
teeth whitening and
you can have it before anyone you know!

Arm yourself with everything you need to know about *healthy* teeth whitening with *The Teeth Whitening Cure.*

CHAPTER 50
THE PERFECT CURE
FOR BLEACH FEVER

THE TROUBLE WITH
TEETH WHITENING PRODUCTS

Even if you're using the best teeth whitening products in the world, your'e still not getting complete whitening support.

So, if you're suffering from yellowing stained teeth, sensitive teeth, bleeding gums, gingivitis, tooth decay, tartar, burning gums, loose teeth, or you just 'can't chew" certain foods...

READ THIS NOW!

Because I've got a breakthrough for you that goes way beyond
the power of teeth whitening gels alone...
at a price that won't make your teeth cry!

A special report by Dr. Lester Sawicki

Dear Friends in Search of Complete and Natural Oral Health,

If there's one thing that makes my teeth grind, it's tall-talking claims for teeth whitening products. And if you suffer any kind of yellow teeth, I'm sure you've seen plenty of hype for teeth whitening gels and strips.

These "miracle solutions" are supposed to solve all the problems of yellow teeth by drowning your teeth in a toxic sea of bleaching chemicals—you know, those *yucky* gel trays and strips of gunk you can't help but swallow into your stomach.

Maybe you're one of the many who have paid a small fortune for teeth whitening products, hoping to banish your yellow teeth. You rip open the box with eager anticipation ... mold the trays ... squirt the gel ... stick on the strips ... *and nothing happens.*

Don't get me wrong. I *do like* teeth whitening and I've been telling my patients to use whitening products for years. But the simple fact is ...

Bleach gels and strips are too measly to tackle it all!

Why? Because, first of all, if you want to brighten and lighten your teeth into a more natural glamorous smile, you also have to strengthen your teeth and gums. The two go hand-in-hand. Bright smiles are astounding, but doing it in a healthy way is more complex than you think. Consider what can happen ...

FIRST, tooth decay—try to whiten your teeth if there is a cavity and the *"electric shock"* will bring *screaming tears of pain* running down your cheeks ...

SECOND, ghost teeth—bleach your teeth *TOO MUCH* and you'll end up with an *"eery bluish"* translucent smile that dentists call ghost teeth.

THIRD, toxic gels—the American Dental Association petitioned the Federal Drug Administration to begin classifying unsafe, irritating, and potentially caustic bleaching chemicals because teeth whitening/bleaching materials are not risk-free.

Getting the picture? Healthy teeth whitening depends on a system that works in harmony with your mouth ...

**But most teeth whitening products
ignore ALL THREE ISSUES
which must be solved to
protect and support your health...**

Which leaves you abandoned and lost without complete healthy teeth whitening!

But not for long. I've got a brand-new breakthrough book that can give you the information needed to take care of **ALL 3** hot spots. I call it *The Teeth Whitening Cure*. And this "miracle book" is about to become your new best friend.

Let me explain...

FIRST, IT SHOWS YOU THE QUICKEST and *most effective way* to stop and prevent tooth decay for just pennies a day.

There is a "little secret" the dental profession has been hiding from you and finally, due to the efforts of a few brave dentists, the secret is out... **tooth decay is caused by acids**... to stop and prevent tooth decay all you have to do is neutralize the acids in your mouth... *fast*... and with one *solid knock-out punch*!

Inside my book you'll discover a way to stop dead any tooth decay germs that might be eating away your tooth enamel... without having to deal with potentially harmful fluoride products that most big, fat cat corporate toothpaste companies try to sell you. Solve the tooth decay issue and you won't have to worry about electric shocks during teeth whitening.

SECOND, GHOST TEETH won't be a problem... if you go *slow and safe*. The trouble is most teeth whitening companies never mention this unsightly side effect because they want you to use and buy as much of their product as you can afford... to make their gold filled pockets even richer with corporate sales bonuses.

Your smarter than that and I know you don't want to "bail out" a tooth whitening conglomerate with your hard earned money. That's why I went out of my way to include this vital information in my book...in your best interest...and to save you tons of money!

THIRD, TOXIC GEL is a hot news item you'll be reading more of. Even the American Dental Association and the Federal Drug Administration are becoming worried about the hazards of swallowing, absorbing, and over use of potentially toxic chemicals found in teeth whitening products. Teeth whitening giant corporations sure aren't the ones bringing up these frightful warnings because they know you would never buy their formulas if you knew.

This is serious business. Why take chances with YOUR health and life? *The Teeth Whitening Cure* has more than several chapters on this topic alone...and I wouldn't do ANY bleaching without first reading its potentially *life saving* information!

So at long last, you can relax and...

**...let *The Teeth Whitening Cure* rescue you
with powerful answers to these 3 hot issues...
...AND MORE!...**
**...so that you'll finally know all you need to know
about teeth whitening.**

AND all of this for a fraction of what you'd pay for over the counter formulas that don't even work! And because I've included so much information about teeth bleaching, in one book, that you can't find anywhere else...without exotic-sounding claims that can't be fulfilled... I'm going to guarantee that this is the best deal you'll ever get for your money. In fact...

The Teeth Whitening Cure is the Perfect Cure for Bleach Fever!

This book is "The Real Missing Link" that can help you achieve an outstanding natural, bright smile... and *better health!*

And I also promise that by using the tons of information you'll read in this book you'll feel better, smile stronger, and give your aura a more energized sexy look.

Best of all, after reading my book—you'll understand how much better you can feel and you'll start looking forward to your next bleaching experience!

The Teeth Whitening Cure and all the helpful tips you'll find in it is about to become your new best friend!

CHAPTER 51
YOUR SOUL VACCINATION AGAINST BLEACH FEVER

From the desk of

Lester Sawicki, D.D.S.
The Smile Power Coach

Dear Health-Conscious Friend,

There are many teeth whitening products that CLAIM to give you a whiter brighter smile, but I haven't found one with just the right formula and dosage your teeth REALLY need for brightness, health, and fitness!

That's why I want to tell you about my book, *The Teeth Whitening Cure.* It reveals the first **Safe** and **Natural** whitening system I've found that offers concentrated whitening AND strengthening in the RIGHT amount just for YOU!... AND... it's **HEALTHY!**

My system gives you the **exact** whitening formula for you and your smile. AND it offers **extra** protection against tooth decay and gum disease... PLUS... no more tears of agony because of cold sensitive teeth!

The Natural Bright Teeth Detox may be your most important 'vitamin' for health and fitness. Very few glamour "smile makeovers" do it right. Their bleaching gels push double, triple, and even quadruple doses of potentially toxic bleach ingredients to get an artificial 'whiter than snow' smile that rarely beautifies nor complements your skin tone. It's an exercise in sheer vanity AND NOT good for your health. You're smarter than that!

We should Brighten our Smile for POWER
in a <u>Healthy Way</u>

Enjoy a beautiful, glamorous, and more NATURAL smile that nature intended just for you. Smile STRONG, BRIGHT and TALL...**AND** feel FIT!...with the help of just "one little secret"...

...AND you won't end up with over whitened 'ghost teeth'... AND don't be surprised if you're suddenly more self-confident, sleep and feel better, and stay more alert...AND all you've done is whiten and DETOX your teeth...PLUS...after you detox your teeth you'll feel a **boost** of ENERGY...You'll have a more natural, brighter smile...AND even find a bounce in your step.

Man SMILING BRIGHT should be man
intensely ALIVE!

Association Press News: <u>Safety Alert</u>!
Did you know?...the American Dental Association petitioned the Federal Drug Administration to begin classifying unsafe, irritating, and potentially caustic bleaching chemicals because teeth whitening/bleaching materials are not risk-free.

Put the brakes on yellowing teeth and throw away your potentially toxic bleaching gels. Discover little known safe, healthy, and natural smile whitening secrets revealed in my book, *The Teeth Whitening Cure.*

Scientists are finding more suspicious connections between cardiovascular disease, diabetes, cancer, and gum health. That's why my book exposes the potentially **toxic** dangers of today's bleaching gels and gives you essential support in the right dosage and form to **naturally** lighten your teeth while increasing your tooth, gum, and total fitness. Everything you need for strong CAVITY FREE teeth, HEALTHIER gums, enhanced cardiovascular support with disease prevention... AND a Bright Smile!

Everyone knows minerals are good for your teeth. Studies have linked too little minerals and too much acid with cavities and sensitive teeth. The research shows that replenishing your mineral levels can not only relieve and prevent cold sensitive teeth, it even prevents jaw muscle fatigue associated with TMJ pain. Yet most teeth whitening gels, strips, liquids, creams, pastes, and applicators give you **DIDDLY** amounts or the **WRONG** kind. That's why I made sure my teeth detox gives you ALL the miracle minerals your teeth need, as well as your muscles and bones.

PLUS, you'll discover **three superhero nutrients** that make all the difference to healthy, natural relief for cold sensitive teeth. With these 3 magic bullets you'll never again waste your hard earned money on artificial, chemically 'frankentainted' desensitizing toothpastes and rinses.

Hold On! This is too important! I won't make you wait until your book arrives in the mail. Here it is—**FREE!**—the three supercharged nutrients that help with sensitive teeth are:

- Magnesium
- Silica
- Strontium

As an extra freebie, I also want you to know scientists are finding that magnesium, silica, and strontium also increase bone mass, density, and strength.

But its not just the natural ingredients that make my Teeth Whitening Detox different from any other whitening and bleaching system... see how safe and easy it can be to enjoy feeling bright, strong, smiling teeth. AND you can do it for *much* less than your dentist prescribed products.

But despite all of this great research and news, most people aren't being told about safe natural ways to whiten and strengthen teeth in a healthier way. Which is why I feel exceptionally good about giving you a book with all this vital information.

Finally, the whole nine yards of smile-building support all in one book! Everything you need to know for strong teeth, a healthier body, and a sexy natural brite smile.

See how easy it can be to enjoy great-feeling, gorgeous strong teeth!

Be More—Feel Better—Smile Longer

Get the Teeth Whitening Cure and see for yourself how easily the right combination of nutrition and bleaching protocol can keep your teeth strong, bright, and healthy!

Experience the Grand Ultimate Teeth Whitening System as described in my book, *The Teeth Whitening Cure*, that has giant corporate 'fat cat' makers of bleaching gels and strips crying "Boo hoo, No Fair! … It's Safer and Healthier!"

The proof on these smile-enhancing secrets is going to knock the teeth bleaching "nuts" right out of their bleach trays!

P.S. It's scientifically proven—your smile has POWER. If you follow the guidelines revealed in my breakthrough book, you are doing all you can to develop your Smile Power—many times more than a lot of dentists offer in their high tech office. You are actually ensuring that you get the longest life and best use from the only teeth you'll ever have.

This book offers interesting surprises and remarkable fascinations for men and women that don't want to quit smiling and playing throughout life. It provides the most effective hidden secrets to optimal healthy teeth and natural smile brightening so YOU can stay at the peak of vibrant excellent health. They *do* work as I've described them—not always, not for everyone all the time, but often enough that I readily recommend them and use them myself.

I realize you are looking for results and I believe *The Teeth Whitening Cure* is the BEST book available to you and is a reliable guide to the best smile whitening and detoxing system in the emerging field of cosmetic dentistry.

Hurry, get your copy TODAY!

CHAPTER 52
EVEN DENTISTS MAY BE SPEECHLESS!

WHEN YOU NEED IT MOST...
The Teeth Whitening Cure **is Here...**
with a *remedy so powerful*
Even DENTISTS May Be Speechless!

JUST IMAGINE... the stunned look on your dentist's face when he announces,

"I can't find a trace of gum disease. Your burning bleeding gums and deep gum pockets have completely stabilized."

Dr. Sawicki searched the most brilliant medical and dental minds on the planet working day and night for one purpose:

To discover the underground cures you need most.

The ones your dentist likely doesn't know a thing about. (It's not his fault. These breakthroughs have been covered up by the PR Machines of the triad family of Big Pharma, Medical and Dental Associations. The ones you'll never hear about on the evening news... or read about in the daily paper.

No, you'll find the latest and most important medical and dental breakthroughs from only one source: *The Teeth Whitening Cure.*

The Only Complete Collection of Natural Cures for:

Tooth Decay

Gum Disease

Teeth Whitening

...without the harmful side effects of prescription medications, fluoride and chemicals—or their exorbitant costs.

It's all here...only the best, natural remedies...with all the details on your body's innate ability to heal itself.

There's a whole lot more, but you can find all the details in *The Teeth Whitening Cure.*

Only the BEST discoveries—now in one book.

Dr. Sawicki is the only dentist that has the inside story on Bleach Fever and why it's a hidden but rapidly growing epidemic...and mainstream's best answer is to watch it grow into a pandemic situation. In fact, they act as if they are even supporting the spread—to further line their pocket books with more green stuff.

But with the information revealed in the Teeth Whitening Cure, you can finally access the "real" answers for Bleach Fever with the latest breakthroughs. Dr. Sawicki let's you in on little known secrets where the power of natural medicine never ceases to amaze...

...Your Soul Vaccination Against Bleach Fever!

Challenge Yourself to Realize
Excellent Physical and Oral Health and...
Reveal Your
TRUE INNER SMILE!

<u>BELIEVE</u> that Art, Science, and Nature can give you a GORGEOUS SMILE!

Purify Your Body
Brighten Your Smile
Balance Your Life

Are You Enjoying Life?

Getting a little Older Doesn't mean giving up the Spice of Life. Anti-aging miracles are here giving you the means to kick up a Healthy, Active Lifestyle. Experts in anti-aging remedies can help you turn back the clock to a time when you were Living High Performance.

You were Born to Be Forever Healthy!

Dr. Sawicki recognizes that Modern medicine has ignored our biological past. <u>That is a mistake</u>. This mistake has led us down a path where we have come to believe only the pharmaceutical industry holds the keys to our health. YOU were born to be healthy—a state that should <u>not</u> depend on drugs.

"I believe we need to start over and give the American people an open and straightforward solution that tackles the real problems of a complete oral health care system."

—Lester Sawicki, D.D.S.

END BONUS CHAPTERS: PART 2

THE TEETH WHITENING CURE

BIOGRAPHY

Dr. Lester Sawicki is an independent general dentist, practicing for more than 33 years. During the first 10 years of his career he directed a very successful practice in the Chicago area and since that time, has sustained recognition in Illinois, Pennsylvania, Texas, Nevada, New Jersey, Alabama, and Puerto Rico. Dr. Sawicki has contributed his knowledge and expertise to nearly 100 dental practices throughout the United States. In 1983, he began studying nutrition and alternative health, and since 2004 has been devoted to intensive research into the relationship between whole body detoxification and longevity. Dr. Sawicki's personal interests include martial arts and meditation. For 20 years he has been a practicing student of Tai Chi, having met many Tai Chi and Chi Kung Masters both in the United States and China. His home is in Austin, Texas.